The Cleveland Clinic Guide to

SLEEP
DISORDERS

Also in the *Cleveland Clinic Guide* Series

The Cleveland Clinic Guide to Arthritis
The Cleveland Clinic Guide to Heart Attacks
The Cleveland Clinic Guide to Menopause
The Cleveland Clinic Guide to Thyroid Disorders

The Cleveland Clinic Guide to

SLEEP DISORDERS

Nancy Foldvary-Schaefer, MD

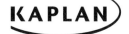

KAPLAN

PUBLISHING

New York

Artwork is reprinted with the permission of The Cleveland Clinic Center for Medical Art & Photograph © 2009.

Published by Kaplan Publishing, a division of Kaplan, Inc.
1 Liberty Plaza, 24th Floor
New York, NY 10006

Library of Congress Cataloging-in-Publication Data
Foldvary-Schaefer, Nancy.
   The Cleveland Clinic guide to sleep disorders / Nancy Foldvary-Schaefer.
   p. cm.
   Includes bibliographical references and index.
   ISBN 978-1-4277-9957-9 (alk. paper)
   1. Sleep disorders--Popular works. I. Title.
   RC547.F65 2009
   616.8'498--dc22

                                        2008049179

10 9 8 7 6 5 4 3 2 1

ISBN-13: 978-1-4277-9957-9

Kaplan Publishing books are available at special quantity discounts to use for sales promotions, employee premiums, or educational purposes. Please email ⟨ **3 1232 00898 2995** ⟩er or for more information at *kaplanpubl* ⟩plan Publishing, 1 Liberty Plaza, 24th Floor, New York, NY 10006.

To Errol Schaefer,
my husband and best friend

and to
Isabela Schaefer,
our ever-smiling daughter

Contents

Introduction

You can't escape references to sleep in modern culture. Terminology and slang related to sleep permeate our language: all-nighters, nightcaps, catnaps, night owls, sleeper movies. Our culture is ever curious about the importance of sleep, even while we search for ways to make the most of our waking hours.

Recent research reminds us of the importance of adequate sleep, the consequences of sleep deprivation, and the impact of sleep disorders on the quality of our lives. Sleep loss affects our mental and physical well-being, interpersonal relationships, and performance behind the wheel, at school, and on the job. And sleep disorders contribute to a variety of medical conditions, including high blood pressure, cardiac arrhythmias, diabetes, and obesity, to name a few. A good night's sleep is critical for a healthy, happy life.

But sleep deprivation has evolved into an epidemic of sorts. If you're like me and most Americans, you have experienced the effects of sleep deprivation or know someone with a sleep disorder. The corporate world pressures us to conform to rigorous schedules. We overprogram ourselves, jamming our days with professional, extracurricular, family, and social activities. We teach our children to do the same, encouraging back-to-back after-school activities that book their free time well into the evening hours. Popular culture has responded to our lack of sleep with solutions to keep us awake, among them the coffee-shop revolution and a wide selection of energy drinks. It's no wonder we are running on empty, building up a sleep deficit as we go through our busy days.

Reflecting these trends, sleep medicine has grown into an established medical specialty, and more people than ever before are turning to sleep specialists and sleep disorders centers for answers. Since I began treating patients with sleep disorders nearly 15 years ago, America has witnessed an explosive growth in the number of physicians choosing sleep as a specialty and an equally impressive proliferation of accredited sleep laboratories. Today we know that sleep affects virtually every aspect of life and interrelates with many disciplines in medicine. As one of the body's basic needs, sleep is responsible for restoring and preserving our health. This book is dedicated to the thousands of men, women, and children with sleep problems whom I have met and treated over the years and who have taught me so much of what I now know about sleep medicine.

If you've picked up this book, you are or someone you love is probably suffering from the effects of inadequate or unrefreshing sleep. Maybe your partner snores horribly, keeping you up for hours if you don't fall asleep first. Or perhaps you lay awake for hours each night for no apparent reason, unable to fall asleep despite a deep feeling of exhaustion (I've done this myself many nights!). Your child might complain of waking up several times a night, or of daytime tiredness.

In these pages, I'll introduce you to the field of sleep medicine, explain the importance of sleep, and give you a glimpse of what sleep testing is all about. Through case histories of some of my own patients, I'll illustrate several of the most common sleep disorders: Obstructive sleep apnea, narcolepsy, psychophysiological insomnia, delayed sleep phase syndrome, sleep terrors and sleepwalking, restless legs syndrome, and REM sleep behavior disorder. And I'll offer pearls and words of caution about treatments that will help you get the z's you need. Above all, I hope to show you that you are not alone.

A book, however, is not a substitute for seeing a doctor. If you suspect that you or a loved one has a sleep disorder, I hope this volume guides you toward the attention you should receive to treat your condition. Because everyone deserves a good night's sleep.

Sweet dreams.

Nancy Foldvary-Schaefer, D.O.
Director
Cleveland Clinic Sleep Disorders Center
Neurological Institute

Associate Professor of Medicine
Cleveland Clinic Lerner College of Medicine of Case Western
    Reserve University
www.clevelandclinic.org/sleep

Chapter 1

Sleep: What It Is and Why You Need It

To achieve the impossible dream, try going to sleep.
—Joan Klempner

Most of us who complain of sleep problems are armed with excuses for our lack of z's.

A worrywart restlessly pores over a mental to-do list: *How am I going to finish this project tomorrow? What did he mean when he said that in the meeting? Am I spending enough time with my children?*

A stubborn professional justifies sleep deficiency as a personality trait: *I've never slept that well anyway. I'm lucky to get six hours.*

Or there's the anthem of the ambitious—more coffee, less sleep: *I'll sleep when I'm dead. Why waste time in bed?*

Chronic nonsleepers often attribute their wakefulness to normal behavior for any "night person." But when we lose sleep, we risk our health. And just as serious are the cases of people who sleep all night but still drag through the day, exhausted. Job performance drops, they doze off during meetings, and they depend on stimulants to restore their energy so they can spend time with family in the evenings. Sleep disorders affect how we feel both at night and during the day.

Sleep isn't a luxury; it is a necessity. Those hours of lost sleep add up to a greater health deficit than many might realize. We need sleep so we can restore nutrients, replenish the spirit, and refresh the mind. Hidden health hazards accumulate during periods of sleeplessness, and they can't be covered up with concealer or reversed with caffeine.

Sleep ranks in importance with diet and exercise, yet many Americans are sleep-deprived—70 million of us, to be exact. The number of people with sleep disorders climbs steadily each year, but we continue to regard sleep as extracurricular and optional.

This attitude is dangerous. And sometimes, the side effects from disrupted sleep are extreme.

Take José, for example.

José

During my very first week working as a sleep specialist, José, 44, hobbled into my office. His leg was broken, but he didn't sustain the injury from sports or anything of the kind. Instead, this father had jumped out of his third-floor bedroom window while sleepwalking. He was escaping a "house fire," he told me, still visibly shaken. Fortunately, he didn't "save" his 3-year-old son, who was sleeping soundly in an adjacent room—though apparently he had tried to do just that. Instead of grabbing the boy, he had tossed a bedside lamp out the window before taking his own plunge. José thought he must have mistaken the lamp for his boy, who normally shared the bed with him and his wife, Mary.

José's broken leg was a wake-up call to a serious sleep disorder.

After the incident, José's wife, Mary, decided that the family needed a new sleeping arrangement. Now, she and their son wish José a goodnight from the safety of the family's spare bedroom. Once inside, Mary locks the windows and door.

"I hate doing this," Mary tells José every night.

Terrified of what might happen if he sleepwalks again, Mary has begged José to see a doctor.

Four percent of the population sleepwalks, but José's activity is more severe than most. More common, perhaps, are situations like John and Barb's.

John and Barb

John and Barb have shared a bed for 18 years. He stretches out on the left; she curls up on the right. He unwinds to the droning noise of the 11 o'clock news; she retires with a best-seller. John rarely lasts through the first commercial break before dozing off, but Barb's reading light might burn past midnight if she's reading a page-turner. He falls asleep on his back; she prefers her side.

They've drifted off like this every night, their routine predictable and comfortable.

During the past year, however, their nighttime ritual has evolved into a frustrating struggle for Barb. A light sleeper, she now falls asleep next to a snoring engine. Minutes after John's head hits the pillow, his mouth drops open and his labored breathing escalates into a loud purr. Before long, he erupts, blasting like a foghorn.

John's episodes worsened over time. But when Barb tells him, "You were really roaring last night," John is surprised. It's only when he finds Barb asleep on the couch in the morning that he realizes his snoring is disruptive.

Doesn't everyone have trouble sleeping once in a while?

Perhaps you aren't like Barb, lying awake at night listening to a snoring bed partner, and you probably aren't mobile at midnight like José. But most of us will experience a string of sleepless nights at some point in our lives—times when our minds simply won't turn off and our thoughts race faster during every minute we spend watching the clock or staring at the ceiling.

If you're generally a comfortable sleeper, a rare night of fitful sleep gives you a taste of how the other camp copes. You might recognize the morning ritual: The alarm clock squawks way too early, and your subsequent drowsiness and "wrong-side-of-the-bed" mood persist, even after several cups of your caffeine of choice.

Imagine a week of wake-up calls like this. Or a month. Or a lifetime.

If you recognize this as your morning scenario, you're not alone. Two-thirds of Americans experience sleep problems at least a few nights a week, according to the 2008 Sleep in America Poll conducted by the National Sleep Foundation, and an astonishing 44 percent reported sleep problems every night or every other night. Children, who are as overprogrammed and stressed as their adult counterparts, also suffer from lack of sleep. Their restlessness takes a toll on caregivers, who can lose up to 200 hours of sleep each year tending to children's nighttime awakenings, the poll reports.

The Importance of Sleep

A good night's sleep is critical to our mental, emotional, and physical health. Not sleeping affects every facet of life, including relationships, work, education, appetite, motivation, and more. In turn, certain medical conditions cause sleep problems. Those diagnosed with conditions such as heart failure, arthritis, heartburn, and epilepsy are less likely to sleep well, and overweight individuals are at higher risk for sleep apnea.

It's clear that we need a good night's sleep. Why, then, is that so impossible for some of us to achieve?

What is sleep, anyway?

Sleep—what it is and what it is not—has stumped the world's greatest thinkers. Early writers and poets pondered this curious state of being, attempting to decipher its relationship to dreaming and death. Sleep plays starring roles in science fiction as well as the stories we grew up reading—at bedtime, ironically.

Sleeping Beauty was cast under a spell that would allow her to awake from an ageless sleep with a kiss from her true love. Rip Van Winkle rested for 20 years. Washington Irving enticed readers with a dreamscape called Sleepy Hollow, where spellbound villagers walked in reverie in the sequestered glen. The Sleepy Hollow Boys, as they were called, heard music and voices in the air, fell into trances, and saw ghosts, including the notorious Headless Horseman.

In his 1834 book *The Philosophy of Sleep*, Robert MacNish mused that sleep was a subconscious middle ground:

Sleep is the intermediate state between wakefulness and death; wakefulness being regarded as the active state of all the animal and intellectual functions, and death as that of their total suspension.

Sleep puzzled people in prehistoric, biblical, and later eras. Dreams, nightmares, and the circadian rhythms of the human body enthralled our ancestors long before science and medicine evolved and research produced data about "normal" sleep cycles (this information wouldn't surface until the 1950s). Distinctions among states of quiescence (coma, stupor, intoxication, hypnosis, and hibernation) were nonexistent. Sleep meant the brain was "off," and when sensory stimulation bombarded the brain, the sleeper woke up.

Then the question of sleep flip-flopped.

"It is perhaps not sleep that needs to be explained, but wakeful-ness," wrote Nathaniel Kleitman in *Sleep and Wakefulness* in 1939. Soon after, scientists studied electrical activity in the brain and discovered the clear, repetitive brain-wave patterns that constitute a sleep cycle. Sleep research progressed during World War II to animal studies, which led to explanations of rapid eye movement (REM) sleep. Sigmund Freud piqued public interest in dreams and

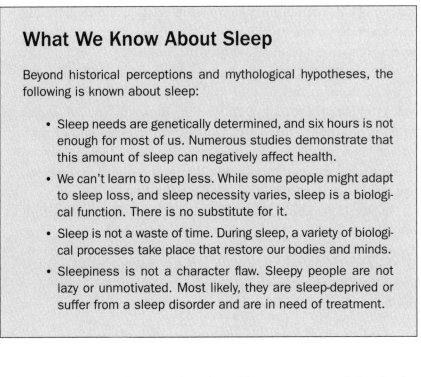

What We Know About Sleep

Beyond historical perceptions and mythological hypotheses, the following is known about sleep:

- Sleep needs are genetically determined, and six hours is not enough for most of us. Numerous studies demonstrate that this amount of sleep can negatively affect health.

- We can't learn to sleep less. While some people might adapt to sleep loss, and sleep necessity varies, sleep is a biological function. There is no substitute for it.

- Sleep is not a waste of time. During sleep, a variety of biological processes take place that restore our bodies and minds.

- Sleepiness is not a character flaw. Sleepy people are not lazy or unmotivated. Most likely, they are sleep-deprived or suffer from a sleep disorder and are in need of treatment.

sparked more sophisticated studies of brain activity and sleep's relationship to psychology.

Sleep history is steeped in mythology, and the study of sleep and dreams still leaves doctors with unanswered questions. Sleep research has pieced together decades of experiments, debunked historical beliefs of what sleep is, and shown that sleep disorders interfere with wakefulness and are indeed a health hazard.

The Basic Anatomy of Sleep

Bodies naturally maintain an internal equilibrium; this is called *homeostasis.* Just as our stomach growls when we feel hunger pangs, and our throat is dry when we are thirsty, our body shuts down when we are tired. We have a homeostatic drive to sleep. Our brain tells us when it's time for lights out.

Our "sleep switch" is located in the hypothalamus of the brain; the front regulates sleep, the back is the wakefulness center. But a variety of other areas within the brain, ranging from brain stem nuclei (collections of brain cells) to structures in the cerebral hemispheres, are also involved in promoting sleep and wakefulness. Neurons in these regions interact with each other; some inhibit sleep-promoting neurons during the day, while others collect in the brain during wakefulness and eventually promote sleep at night. This "circuit" within the brain helps the body sustain a sleep-wake balance that is as necessary as food and drink.

Working in tandem with this drive is the circadian clock, which we will discuss further in chapter 11. The circadian clock is regulated by a specific group of brain cells in the hypothalamus. The circadian clock is synchronized with the external environment to coordinate sleep and wakefulness.

What is a sleep disorder?

Sleep disorders are disturbances that affect normal patterns of sleep and wakefulness. There are more than 80 sleep disorders, and they affect everyone from babies to the elderly. Many people who suffer from sleep disorders do not seek the help they need.

Together, the circadian clock's alerting signal and our homeostatic drive to sleep tell our bodies when to sleep and when to wake up. Sleep disorders arise when these messages are confused, out of sync, or disrupted.

Do men and women suffer from the same sleep problems?

Although men and women share common sleep problems, some problems are more prevalent in one gender. Some problems are specific to age groups, such as teens, children, and the elderly. The following are some sleep generalizations for each group:

Men

General Attitudes: *Sleep gets in the way of work . . . . If I'm sleeping, I'm unproductive . . . . Lazy people need more sleep—I've got too much to do and far too many responsibilities . . . . My wife complains I snore like a freight train, but I sleep just fine . . . .*

Sleep obstacles: Some people sacrifice downtime in the evening to work longer and harder so they can get ahead. Rather than reading a book or doing other activities to unwind, they boot up their laptops and plug away into the wee hours. It can take hours to free your mind after an exhausting day at work. Stop number crunching and strategic planning before midnight, and allow your mind to slow down.

According to the 2008 Sleep in America Poll, 30 percent of respondents said they work 50 hours or more per week. Men, in particular, were likely to fall into this group. Further, men were more likely to be shift workers, work six or seven days a week, and be obese, setting the stage for sleep deprivation. Lack of sleep can hinder work performance and increase the chance of occupational injuries and motor vehicle accidents. Researchers have also found crucial links between sleep loss and major medical conditions, such as obesity and diabetes, making their treatment more challenging.

In addition to work, men's schedules are packed with home-improvement projects, working out at the gym, participating in sports, volunteering for civic groups, spending time with family, and other personal pursuits. When life changes enter the picture (such as marriage, a new baby, a new job, a move, or a death in the family), men tend to bottle up feelings rather than release them by venting to friends and family. When men reach a breaking point, the worry jar almost always opens when the lights are out. And when you can't solve problems, they become more dramatic and urgent, growing from a small "what-if" to a crisis.

Women

General Attitudes: *How can I balance family, work, and friends? . . . . I feel as if my life is pulled in so many directions, that's all I can think about when I wake up at night . . . . My body is telling me it needs rest, but my mind won't slow down . . . .*

Sleep Obstacles: Some of the sleep challenges confronting women are related to hormonal changes during pregnancy, menstruation, and menopause. Postpartum depression can also trigger insomnia in some women. As a woman progresses through the stages of her life, she is prone to sleeping less or waking up more often during the night. After menopause, women are more likely to be diagnosed with sleep disorders such as obstructive sleep apnea.

Women of all ages experience sleep problems, but the problems change and increase in severity across the lifespan. According to the 2007 National Sleep Foundation poll, 60 percent of American women said they get a good night's sleep only a few nights per week or less. Regardless of whether a woman is a working mother, or a homemaker, young or old, a lack of sleep affects virtually every aspect of her life, leaving her tired and stressed as she juggles family, social, and work-related commitments.

Teenagers

General Attitudes: *With school, friends, and sports, I don't have time to sleep . . . . I have to wake up for school so early, but I'm not ready to go to bed early at night, so it's hard to stay awake during class . . . . I'm a night person . . . .*

Sleep Obstacles: Time might be the greatest challenge for today's teenagers, and sleep loses out to school, sports, jobs, and social activities. A recent survey by the American Academy of Sleep Medicine shows that only 15 percent of teenagers regularly get the nine hours of sleep they need each night. That means 85 percent of 13- to 19-year-olds are running on empty. Twenty-six percent of young people clock six or fewer hours under the covers each night.

As the teenage body works through puberty, it experiences a shift in circadian rhythm (the body's 24-hour clock). Although younger children are apt to feel tired at 8 or 9 P.M., teens' circadian clocks shift to a later sleep time of 10 or 11 P.M. At the same time these changes are taking place, school starts early in the morning followed by extracurricular activities that carry on late into evening. Sleep is just another elective.

Children and the elderly And too, attitudes about sleep and associated obstacles occur across the lifetime. Without adequate sleep, a healthy, happy baby can develop into a problem child. A child's disposition often is the first indication of sleep deficit. Rather than being lighthearted, smiling, and energetic, a tired child is cranky and hyperactive.

As people age, their sleep habits change significantly. For people over age 65, it is important to distinguish between what is normal and what symptoms are signs of a sleep disorder. (Both age groups are covered more thoroughly in chapter 12.)

The dangers of sleep deprivation

Sleep deprivation has become one of the most important and unrecognized public health issues of modern times. Lack of sleep is often chronic and a result of the excessive social and work demands of modern life, coupled with poor sleep habits. Daytime sleepiness is the primary result, but there is a host of other symptoms that accompany sleep deprivation, including fatigue, low energy, poor concentration, inattention, and irritability. Nighttime sleep is often shorter in duration than expected, leading to the common habit of sleeping in on weekends to "catch up." Sleep loss of this nature affects at least one-third of normal adults and is especially severe in night-shift workers. Sleep fragmentation due to repeated arousals from sleep, as seen in sleep apnea and other disorders, results in similar neurobehavioral consequences and decrements in performance.

The detrimental effects of sleep deprivation have been studied for more than a century. Some of the effects of severe sleep loss include:

- Sleepiness, especially severe at night, which can be overcome to varying degrees with external stimulation, like physical activity. Brief sleep episodes called *microsleeps*, which are usually imperceptible to the subject, are often evident.

- Mild dysphoria and irritability.

- Impaired performance in tasks requiring close attention, such as balancing a checkbook, but not visually stimulating motor activities, like playing exciting arcade games. Performance can be temporarily improved with motivation and incentives.

- Neurological disturbances including visual illusions and hallucinations, blurred vision, drooping eyelids, disorientation, incoordination, slurred speech, memory lapses, slowed mentation, and difficulty thinking.

Limiting sleep to four to six hours per night over a period of one to two weeks produces significant impairments in cognitive performance and increases daytime sleepiness. These cognitive effects are equivalent to the effect produced by two nights of not sleeping at all. So be on guard, because many people are completely unaware of these impairments.

Mood will be the first to go if you are sleep-deprived. Studies have consistently found that mood is more vulnerable to sleep deprivation than either cognitive or motor skills. Mood ratings of sleep-deprived subjects are more than three standard deviations worse than ratings of non-sleep deprived individuals.

Performance decrements follow. One series of experiments found that the average level of functioning of sleep-deprived subjects was comparable to that of only the 9th percentile of non-sleep-deprived subjects. Generally, the most profound impairments are observed on tasks that are long and monotonous.

The impact of sleep deprivation on performance is particularly relevant in everyday tasks such as driving and in certain occupations where chronic sleep loss is common. The U.S. Department of Transportation identified fatigue as the number one safety problem in transportation operations, costing billions of dollars annually. In June 2003, New Jersey was the first U.S. state to pass legislation prohibiting driving a motor vehicle while impaired by lack of sleep. Impairment in simulated driving tests after modest sleep loss is comparable to impairment produced by alcohol. And the combined effect of sleep restriction and alcohol is a double whammy, even with low alcohol intake and alcohol concentrations below 0.08%, the legal intoxication level in most states. The effects of regular sleep loss on driving are further exacerbated by coexisting disorders like sleep apnea. Treating sleep apnea can reduce the risk of traffic accidents.

Since our propensity to sleep is a balance between sleep debt and level of arousal, it stands to reason that factors that increase arousal can counteract and even mask the effects of sleep deprivation. Physical activity or exercise and stimulant drugs, including caffeine, are common examples. Bright light, noise, and ambient temperature can also help keep you awake. A driving simulator study of radio noise and cold air in sleep-deprived young adults demonstrated improvement in the subjects' perception of sleepiness and a trend toward reduction of "lane-drifting" incidents. The increased alertness was however only marginal and short-lived, and comparatively less effective than a 15-minute nap or a cup of coffee. The take-home message? Do not rely, as many do, on your radio or cell phone to keep you safe behind the wheel when you are tired.

In addition to the adverse consequences of sleep deprivation on psychological and neurological functions, changes involving the cardiovascular, respiratory, endocrine, and immune systems are also observed. Several large studies have found an association between cardiovascular morbidity and chronic sleep restriction. In the Nurses' Health Study, established in 1976 and the most definitive long-term epidemiological studies conducted to date on older women's health, women sleeping less than seven hours per night had an increased risk of coronary events compared to those averaging eight hours. Sleep deprivation has been shown to cause respiratory irregularities in normal infants and adults with obstructive sleep apnea, impaired glucose tolerance, and elevated evening cortisol levels, a hormone that helps the body manage stress. Abnormal thyroid function and growth hormone secretion can also occur. Finally, many people find their immune system breaks down when they've burned the candle at both ends. Colds are more common when we're sleep deprived because our body's ability to ward off infection is diminished.

How to catch up, you ask? The detrimental effects of sleep deprivation seem to reverse after one to three nights of recovery sleep. The good news, if there's anything at all good about it, is that the amount of sleep required to restore your body to its normal self seems to be less than—in fact as little as 25 percent of—the total amount of sleep lost.

Measures to address the potentially devastating effects of the sleep-deprivation epidemic are cropping up everywhere. In the last decade alone, we've seen legislation against drowsy driving, later school start times, and restriction of duty hours for physician trainees, pilots, and interstate truckers. These measures highlight the serious health and socioeconomic consequences of sleep loss in America and in most other industrialized countries.

Sleep: A Billion-Dollar Industry

A quick inventory of over-the-counter sleep aids, products that promise to cure snoring, and herbal remedies indicates that people aren't just talking more about their sleep habits. They're also recognizing that they need sleep and are looking for a cure. Television commercials assure us that we don't have to go another night without it either.

Americans filled more than 44 million prescriptions for sleeping pills in 2007, up from 35 million in 2004, according to data from Verispan, a company that provides market research and sales data on prescription drugs to the health care industry. Consumers spent more than $1 billion during that year, and more than half of the prescriptions were for Ambien, the first of a new generation of sleep aids. According to an analysis by research house Thomson Health care, about 8 percent of the insured population took sleeping pills in 2006, compared with 5 percent in 1998. And adults are not the only ones reaching for a magic bullet. The survey also found a marked increase in the use of sleeping pills by young adults. Sleep drugs are big business, and there is no sign of the trend lulling into "snooze" as we continue to reach for pill-bottle solutions.

Most of us who need a quick pick-me-up turn to caffeine. Stimulants combat the chronic partial sleep deprivation that modern society encourages. The success of Starbucks is due, in part, to our sleep-deprived society. We demand the strong, caffeinated drinks the chain sells—and Starbucks sells lots of them.

At the same time our consumption of sleep aids and stimulants is increasing, more of us—desperate for a good night's sleep—are reserving beds at sleep labs for overnight testing. Today's overnight sleep studies are not reserved only for patients with obstructive sleep apnea. Labs are equipped to test children and to cater to those with special needs.

The number of treatments and testing options available may seem overwhelming, especially to people who are still getting used to the idea that a lack of sufficient, quality sleep can be seriously detrimental to our health. So many of us have gotten used to sleeping less than we might like—and less than our bodies need—that it can be difficult to tell what is just a normal period of bad nights and what may require medical or behavioral treatment. In order to distinguish one situation from the other, let's review the signs that indicate that you might be suffering from a sleep disorder.

Chapter 2

Do I Have a Sleep Disorder?

A ruffled mind makes a restless pillow.
– Charlotte Brontë

Plenty of exhausted people downplay restless nights and drowsy days by attributing sleep loss to environmental distractions. Take Ruth, who tunes into every drip from the faucet, every creak and curious noise. Each tempts her from her bed to check what could be causing such a racket. While tossing and turning, she creates a mental to-do list that keeps her up even later. She eventually falls asleep right before her alarm clock buzzes. Does Ruth suffer from lack of sleep? Sure, she says, blaming her tired eyes on noisy distractions.

Or perhaps you can relate to Les, who crashes into a sleep so deep that even a blaring television doesn't disturb him. Nothing wakes him—not ringing phones, cacophony from the living room, or the 110-pound hound dog that joins him in bed as soon as he crawls under the sheets. Yet Les is chronically sleepy most days, regardless of how long he sleeps at night. If he could curl up on a couch between meetings at the office, he'd fall fast asleep. In fact, that's how he spends most Sundays.

These two scenarios are normal to many people. Les and Ruth might remind you of a spouse or even yourself. And though your symptoms might not match theirs or be nearly as severe, the fact that you suffer through long, tiring days is reason enough to talk to your doctor.

What's the big deal about sleep, anyway?

The loss of sleep is not just a nighttime problem. Sleep is designed to rejuvenate the body so it can function properly during waking hours. Sleep "activity" is just as critical as wakeful activity. The quality time you spend working through various stages of the sleep cycle is just as important to your physical well-being as eating your vegetables and taking 10,000 steps a day for exercise. In addition, sleep loss poses an increased risk for certain ailments, such as metabolic and endocrine disorders like diabetes, and affects mental health as well.

Sleep deficit accumulates over time, and if you experience sleeplessness during several nights each week, it will affect your work (impaired concentration, slowed reaction time, poor performance), relationships (impatience, crankiness, irritable behavior), and safety (driving and workplace accidents).

How do I know if I have a sleep disorder?

How do you know if your wide-awake nights or sleepy days require treatment from a doctor or a sleep medicine specialist? Answering the following questions will determine whether your sleep habits require attention:

- Are you often tired or sleepy during the day?
- Do you snore or is your breathing interrupted during sleep?
- Do you kick or thrash while your sleep?
- Do you have trouble falling or staying asleep?

- Do you have a family history of sleep disorders?
- Do you have an urge to move your legs at night that interferes with your ability to fall asleep?
- Do you experience unusual behaviors while you sleep, such as walking, eating, or acting out dreams, that interfere with sleep quality or have caused injury to yourself or others?
- Do you have irregular or inconsistent sleep and wake-up times? Is your bedroom environment noisy, bright, or uncomfortable?
- Has your sleep problem been present for more than three months?

If you answer "Yes" to any of these questions, the nighttime rituals you have grown used to and eventually accepted as "normal" are potential symptoms of a sleep disorder. The good news: With monitoring and treatment, you could be able to say "Good night"—and mean it.

With the invention of the lightbulb and ready availability of electrical power, sleep loss has become increasingly prevalent in industrialized nations. Air travel across multiple time zones, globalization of commercial markets, shift work, 24-hours services, television and the Internet have all contributed to longer days and a reduction in the time people spend sleeping. For Americans, the mean number of hours of sleep has fallen steadily in the past century from about 9 hours to about 6.7 hours in 2008 based on the most recent National Sleep Foundation Poll. According to the poll, the average American's workday is 9 hours and 28 minutes long, and two-thirds of us do work-related activities at home outside of regular work hours. The result? Among poll respondents, 29 percent fell asleep or became very sleepy at work during the past month, 36 percent have fallen asleep or nodded off while driving at least once per month during the past year, and 20 percent have lost interest in sex because they are too sleepy.

Red Flag: Sleep Deprivation Signals

If you have been suffering from the following signs of sleep deprivation, make an appointment to see your doctor or a sleep specialist for further evaluation and testing:

- Impaired memory or shortened attention span
- Loss of temper and irritability
- Dozing off or head nodding while you are driving a car or attending a meeting
- Hitting the alarm clock snooze button repeatedly
- Feeling unmotivated or lacking energy to "get going"

The Sleep Cycle and "Normal" Sleep

Identifying what constitutes a "normal" night's sleep can be a challenge. For some, normal is snoring away the first hours of the night, and then tossing and turning until daybreak. Maybe for you, taking hours to fall asleep is part of the routine. You've seen more infomercials than you care to admit and have watched countless reruns.

It's true that sleep is different for each of us. So what is normal? For decades, scientists pondered that question. Sleep research has helped identify what sleep is and how it differs from other states of mind.

After examining records from all-night sleep recordings, researchers noticed a predictable sequence of patterns over the course of a night. Overnight studies (which record a variety of body functions during sleep, including electrical activity in the brain, eye movements, muscle activity, heart rate, breathing effort, airflow through the nose and mouth, and oxygen levels) uncovered what they called the *duality of sleep* or the difference between rapid eye movement (REM) sleep and non-rapid eye movement (NREM) sleep.

What's the difference between REM and NREM sleep?

Rapid eye movement (REM) sleep is a mentally active period during which dreaming and rapid eye movements occur (you can observe this state by watching a sleeping cat) and the skeletal muscles of the body assume a paralyzed state. During NREM sleep, heart rate and breathing slow, and blood pressure decreases, and the body may twitch a few times as one falls asleep. We dream during NREM sleep, too. Non-rapid eye movement (NREM) sleep is divided into three stages, each of which increases in depth until REM sleep begins. Overnight sleep observations demonstrate how sleep normally progresses during the night.

Normal Adult Histogram:

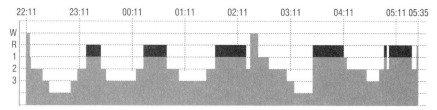

Note: Abundant Stage 3 (deep sleep) in the first half of the night. REM periods (in solid black) progressively increase as the night ensues; one awakening (bathroom break) a little after 2 A.M.

This histogram shows a normal young adult's night of sleep. If you are jolted out of a sound sleep after only a few hours, chances are you have completed only a portion of the full sleep cycle, leaving you deprived of true, sound sleep.

The following histogram depicts the restless night of a patient with insomnia.

Insomnia Histogram:

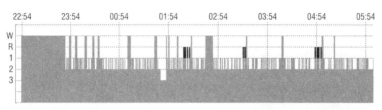

Note: A typical insomniac in a sleep lab experiences a long sleep latency with frequent awakenings and little or no deep sleep (Stage 3) and REM. Similar patterns may be seen in people without insomnia but who have difficulty sleeping because of the laboratory environment.

What does a normal sleep cycle look like?

A sleep period begins with NREM sleep, which usually constitutes 75 to 80 percent of sleep time. NREM sleep is divided into three stages.

- **Stage 1:** 5–10 percent of sleep time.
  Stage 1, also known as drowsiness, is the first and lightest sleep stage.

- **Stage 2:** 30–50 percent of sleep time.
  Stages 1 and 2 are light sleep. Stage 2 follows Stage 1 as one descends into the sleep cycle.

- **Stage 3:** 20–40 percent of sleep time.
  Stages 3 is deep sleep, or slow wave sleep (SWS). Deep sleep refreshes and restores the mind and body.

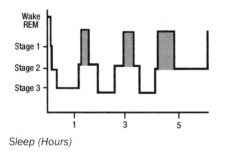

Sleep (Hours)

Shortly after the first SWS period, the body enters REM sleep, which constitutes 20 to 25 percent of sleep time. REM sleep is a mentally active period characterized by bursts of rapid eye movements. During this time, dreaming occurs and brain

When Should I Talk to the Doctor?

One of the primary signals of a sleep disorder is whether the problem (insomnia or sleepiness, for example) adversely affects daytime functioning. We often forget that sleep disorders include problems with wakefulness—in other words, difficulty staying awake despite a seemingly adequate amount of sleep.

Ask yourself the following questions:

- Do you regularly (at least a few times per week) have trouble falling asleep at night?
- Are you sleepy, tired, and lagging most days, despite a good night's sleep?

If the answer to either of these questions is "Yes," it would be a good idea to talk to your doctor about your sleeping habits.

activity increases, as do blood pressure, heart rate, and other body functions when compared to the same rates during SWS periods.

Although the body is paralyzed during REM sleep, brain activity during this time is intense. Scientists have learned that subjects who are awakened during REM sleep remember their dreams, and that dreams vary in length depending on the time of the night in which the REM sleep cycle occurs. A complete sleep cycle generally takes 90 minutes on average. Adults experience four to six sleep cycles during the night.

The research makes clear that REM sleep is evidence that sleep is complex and not a halfway point to coma or death. The discovery of REM sleep in 1953 changed the way that researchers explained sleep. Understanding that the body is not completely "at rest," but instead is recharging, further defines sleep's role in body and health restoration.

What your doctor needs to know

If you're like most people, you probably go to your doctor only when you must. Many of us make the mistake of not being prepared when the doctor enters the room, and we forget to discuss things that do not seem pressing or "life-threatening." Sleep is one of those things. Before your next visit, make an inventory of your sleep habits and complaints and plan to tell your doctor what he or she needs to know.

What is your sleep hygiene like?

Sleep hygiene describes the lifestyle and dietary habits that affect sleep behavior. Most of the concepts are a matter of common sense: avoiding caffeine late in the day, moderating alcohol intake, and creating an inviting environment for sleep (a dark, quiet room is best). (Chapter 8 addresses sleep hygiene more as it relates to insomnia.)

As you consider whether your disruptive sleep behavior is actually a sleep disorder and cause for medical attention, ask yourself these questions pertaining to your sleep hygiene:

- Do you go to bed at the same time every night?
- Do you use the bed for activities like watching television and reading?
- Is your bedroom conducive to sleep?
- Are your sleep patterns the same on weekdays and on weekends?
- Are your waking times irregular?

Recognize the Signs of Drowsy Driving:

- Trouble focusing on the road
- Difficulty keeping the eyes open or closing the eyes at stoplights
- Nodding

You might as well be drunk!

Nine out of ten North American police officers have stopped a driver whom they believed was drunk but turned out to be drowsy, according to the 2004 American Automobile Association Foundation for Traffic Safety Internet Survey. When sleep-deprived drivers get behind the wheel, their motor skills, alertness, and performance are impaired. In fact, researchers have shown that after 17 hours awake, an individual's performance behind the wheel is comparable to how he or she would perform with a blood alcohol concentration of 0.05 percent. After 24 hours awake, performance is comparable to a blood alcohol concentration of 0.1 percent (driving with a level of 0.08 percent or higher is illegal). Drowsiness contributes to 100,000 police-reported crashes annually, according to the U.S. National Highway Traffic Safety Administration.

- Yawning repeatedly
- Drifting from your lane to another one
- Missing signs or exits
- Not remembering driving the last few miles

• • • Fast Fact • • •

According to the 2005 and 2006 *Sleep in America* polls conducted by the National Sleep Foundation:

- 60 percent of drivers admit to driving while they were drowsy during the past year.
- 15 percent of teens in 10th to 12th grades drive drowsy at least *once a week.*
- 33 percent of driver respondents admit to nodding off or falling asleep while driving.
- 4 percent of the drivers had an accident or near accident because they dozed off or were too tired while driving.

• • •

What is your sleep history?

Just as with any other health concern, your doctor will want to get a full description of how you have been sleeping, both recently and in the past. Your physician will gather the information that is necessary to diagnose a potential sleep disorder, to tailor an overnight sleep study so it meets your specific needs, and to designate an appropriate treatment program.

Some sleep centers ask patients to complete a questionnaire about their sleep habits and complaints. This questionnaire provides you with an opportunity to list your primary problem and the related behaviors that affect your ability to sleep soundly, but it is not a surrogate for a one-on-one interview with a sleep specialist.

Starting with basic questions about gender, height, and weight, the sleep history expands into more detailed subjects, such as whether you work a second or third shift, your preferred sleeping position, and whether you take prescription or over-the-counter drugs to help you sleep.

You can expect to discuss the following topics with your physician during a sleep interview:

- Sleep habits
- Daytime sleepiness
- Nighttime behaviors
- Childhood sleep

A sleep interview is the first step toward diagnosing a sleep disorder. Oftentimes, sleep specialists use additional questionnaires to paint a picture of your sleeping habits at night and alertness levels during the day. Your answers allow your sleep patterns to be compared to normal patterns.

The sleep interview is a one-on-one conversation between you and your doctor. Standardized questionnaires that ask you to consider your habits and activities help the doctor determine whether testing in a sleep laboratory is necessary. Many times, the sleep interview alone provides a doctor with enough information to diagnose a sleep disorder and develop a treatment program.

What are your sleep patterns like?

Doctors document sleep patterns by charting activity during a 24-hour period. Your doctor may ask you to keep a sleep log or diary for a week or two, or perhaps longer. Sleep logs help your doctor identify problems such as insufficient sleep as a cause of daytime sleepiness or irregular sleep-wake cycles.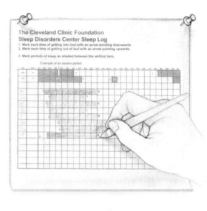

Sleep specialists use a variety of questionnaires that are designed to screen for different sleep, medical, and psychiatric disorders. The questionnaires I find particularly helpful are:

The Epworth Sleepiness Scale This scale asks you to rate how likely you are to fall sleep in certain situations as opposed to just feeling tired. You rate your level of anticipated sleepiness based on your recent past. Even if you have not participated in some of these activities queried in the questionnaire, you are asked to imagine how your body might respond.

The Epworth Sleepiness Scale uses the following scale:

0 = would **never** doze
1 = **slight** chance of dozing
2 = **moderate** chance of dozing
3 = **high** chance of dozing

Situation Chance of Dozing

Situation	Chance of Dozing			
	Never	Slight	Moderate	High
• Sitting and reading				
• Watching television				
• Sitting and inactive in a public place (e.g., a theater or a meeting)				
• Riding as a passenger in a car without a break				
• Lying down to rest in the afternoon when circumstances permit				
• Sitting and talking to someone				
• Sitting quietly after eating a lunch that did not include any alcohol				
• In a car while stopped for a few minutes in traffic				

The eight responses are tallied, producing a score between 0 and 24, with higher scores indicating more significant degrees of sleepiness. A score of 10 or greater is considered abnormal and signifies daytime sleepiness.

The Fatigue Severity Scale This scale asks you to choose a number between 1 and 7 to indicate your level of agreement with each statement (1 = strongly disagree; 7 = strongly agree). It measures the impact of fatigue on how a person functions.

1. My motivation is lower when I am fatigued.
2. Exercise brings on my fatigue.
3. I am easily fatigued.

4. Fatigue interferes with my physical conditioning.
5. Fatigue causes frequent problems for me.
6. My fatigue prevents sustained physical functioning.
7. Fatigue interferes with carrying out certain duties and responsibilities.
8. Fatigue is among my three most disabling symptoms.
9. Fatigue interferes with my work, family, or social life.

The nine responses are tallied with results ranging from 0 to 63. A score of 36 or higher is abnormal, indicating significant functional impairment due to fatigue.

The STOP questionnaire for obstructive sleep apnea This questionnaire consists of four questions:

S: Do you *snore* loudly?
T: Do you often feel *tired*, fatigued, or sleepy during daytime?
O: Has anyone *observed* you stop breathing during sleep?
P: Have you been or are you being treated for high blood *pressure*?

If you answered "Yes" to two or more of the questions, then you are considered at high risk for obstructive sleep apnea (OSA). In the presence of other risk factors for OSA, such as obesity, age over 50, large neck circumference, and male gender, the ability of the STOP questionnaire to predict OSA is even greater.

Patient Health Questionnaire (PHQ-9) This questionnaire is one of several tools that screen for depression, which often accompanies sleep complaints. There are ten questions. Patients choose the response that best describes how often they have been bothered by the following problems during the past two weeks.

1. Little interest or pleasure in doing things:
    0 = Not at all
    1 = Several days
    2 = More than half the days
    3 = Nearly every day

2. Feeling down, depressed, or hopeless:
   0 = Not at all
   1 = Several days
   2 = More than half the days
   3 = Nearly every day

3. Trouble falling or staying asleep, or sleeping too much:
   0 = Not at all
   1 = Several days
   2 = More than half the days
   3 = Nearly every day

4. Feeling tired or having little energy:
   0 = Not at all
   1 = Several days
   2 = More than half the days
   3 = Nearly every day

5. Poor appetite or overeating:
   0 = Not at all
   1 = Several days
   2 = More than half the days
   3 = Nearly every day

6. Feeling bad about yourself or feeling that you are a failure or have let yourself or your family down:
   0 = Not at all
   1 = Several days
   2 = More than half the days
   3 = Nearly every day

7. Trouble concentrating on things, such as reading the newspaper or watching television:
   0 = Not at all
   1 = Several days
   2 = More than half the days
   3 = Nearly every day

8. Moving or speaking so slowly that other people might have noticed. Or the opposite: being so fidgety or restless that you have been moving around a lot more than usual.
   0 = Not at all
   1 = Several days
   2 = More than half the days
   3 = Nearly every day

9. Thoughts that you would be better off dead, or of hurting yourself in some way:
   0 = Not at all
   1 = Several days
   2 = More than half the days
   3 = Nearly every day

10. If you checked off *any* problems, how *difficult* have these problems made it for you to do your work, take care of things at home, or get along with other people?
    0 = Not difficult at all
    1 = Somewhat difficult
    2 = Very difficult
    3 = Extremely difficult

Add the responses of questions 1 through 9 for a total score between 0 and 27. The following cutoff points are used to rate depression severity:

   0–4: None
   5–9: Mild depression
   10–14: Moderate depression
   15–19: Moderately severe depression
   20–27: Severe depression

Your sleep patterns, habits, and behaviors, and how they have changed over time, are the most important part of a sleep evaluation, and they provide critical information that your doctor needs

A to Z's—Some Helpful Terms

Good sleep hygiene: Habits that promote healthy sleep, such as maintaining regular bed times and wake-up times, avoiding caffeine and alcohol before bed, and using your bed only for sleep.

Multiple Sleep Latency Test (MSLT): A daytime test consisting of allowing the patient to take a series of naps during the day at scheduled times in a sleep laboratory following an overnight sleep study. The purpose is to evaluate the complaint of daytime sleepiness.

Polysomnogram (PSG): An overnight sleep study that takes place in a sleep lab.

Sleep latency: How long it takes a person to fall asleep. For example, if your sleep latency is five minutes, you fall asleep easily.

Sleep onset: When a person first falls asleep.

Sleep stages: The sleep cycle comprises three stages of sleep called non-rapid eye movement (NREM) plus rapid eye movement (REM) sleep. We progress through the cycle several times each night

to know. In some cases, the sleep history is all that is needed to diagnose a sleep disorder and develop a treatment plan. This information informs your doctor's determination about what type of testing will best address your needs and the sleep specialist's interpretation of your study. The more information your doctor has about your sleep problem, the better.

Chapter 3

The Sleep Study Experience

A good laugh and a long sleep are the best cures in the doctor's book.

—Irish proverb

Most adults have had difficulty getting a good night's sleep or have experienced daytime sleepiness at some point in their lives. Environmental conditions and life changes that provoke periods of emotional distress—a death in the family, divorce—can trigger a temporary bout of insomnia. Sleep loss to make a deadline may lead to daytime sleepiness or poor performance on the job. This is common, and the problem will resolve once a normal sleep pattern is reestablished.

But what should you do if a few nights of lost sleep multiply into weeks, months, or even years? What about when daytime sleepiness or fatigue occurs even after seemingly good nights of sleep? A sleep disorder can last a short period, or it can develop into a health-threatening illness that affects all aspects of your life.

Getting Professional Help

In order to determine whether your sleep complaint is cause for concern, your doctor will want to collect facts about your sleep-wake patterns and may request that you maintain a log that details time in bed, time asleep, nighttime behavior, and feelings of fatigue or sleepiness during the day (see chapter 2). You may not know the answers to every question a physician asks you about your sleep habits. You might deny snoring until a bed partner complains. You might not realize that you stop breathing in your sleep; you only know that you wake frequently during the night and are tired most days.

If you report excessive daytime sleepiness, your physician will probably recommend an overnight sleep study. Excessive sleepiness almost always signifies a sleep disorder, although medical disorders and medications (including over-the-counter drugs) may contribute to the problem. Patients who experience daytime sleepiness might suffer from such common sleep disorders as insufficient sleep syndrome, sleep apnea, or narcolepsy.

Patients who complain of insomnia generally benefit most from clinical treatment, but sometimes an overnight sleep test can shed new light on their sleep habits. Some insomniacs have false impressions of exactly how many hours they spend sleeping each night. This is called *sleep-state misperception,* and it is common among those with psychophysiological insomnia and insomnia related to psychiatric disorders. A tailored overnight sleep study is another piece of the diagnostic puzzle.

What is a sleep study?

The term *sleep study* refers to a study conducted over the course of one night, and sometimes also during several hours of the ensuing day, that records and evaluates multiple aspects of a patient's sleep. The most common type of sleep study is called a *polysomnogram,* a test conducted during an overnight stay in a sleep lab.

The polysomnogram is a critical tool in evaluating, diagnosing, and treating sleep disorders because it reveals information you probably don't know about your own sleep. Conducted during an eight-hour period, it provides a detailed picture of your sleep-wake patterns over the course of one night. (The test also can take place during the day if a person works third shift or has other special circumstances.)

If you struggle to get a good night's sleep, the thought of checking into a medical facility and tucking into a strange bed in a sterile environment probably doesn't seem like any way to rest easy. Add the wires, monitors, and hardware essential to recording your sleep patterns—as if you will sleep—and you're as likely to doze off in the sleep lab as in the dentist's chair during a root canal, right?

Never fear. Although the study environment is a bit awkward and not as comfortable as your own bed, rest assured that virtually everyone falls asleep during an overnight study. (And if you are have a sleep disorder, you are probably so exhausted that even if you think you won't catch a wink, your body will take advantage of the sleep-friendly environment.)

What does the polysomnogram entail?

During a polysomnogram, a technologist monitors several functions by placing sensors, also known as electrodes, on specific locations on your body. Electrodes aren't painful—although some people compare their removal to the annoyance of ripping off a Band-Aid!

EEG An electroencephalogram records brain-wave activity, which indicates whether a person is awake or asleep and identifies the various stages of sleep (NREM stages 1 through 3 and REM). To gather the data, six to eight (or sometimes more) electrodes are placed at precise locations on the head.

EOG Electro-oculography is the recording of eye movements. Slow eye movements occur during drowsiness, and rapid eye movements take place during REM sleep and wakefulness. Electrodes are attached to the skin at the outside corner of each eye to collect this information.

EMG In electromyography, electrodes are placed over muscles to record movements and muscle tone. In overnight sleep studies, EMG electrodes are placed on the chin to detect changes in muscle tone, which, in turn, helps determine sleep stages. During REM sleep, for example, the tone of skeletal muscles is very low as the body completely relaxes and, in fact, is paralyzed. (At the same time, eye movement activity speeds up, as detected by the EOG.) EMG electrodes are also placed over specified muscles in the arms and legs, in particular over the shins, to measure periodic and random leg movements, which can interfere with sleep quality.

EKG An electrocardiogram is recorded during overnight sleep tests through sensors placed on the chest. The sensors measure heart rate and rhythm during sleep and wakefulness. If a patient suffers from sleep apnea and stops breathing—or has *apneas*—for ten seconds or longer at a time, his or her heart rate can slow down, speed up, or fall into an abnormal rhythm.

Respiration Airflow from the nose and mouth is recorded to identify periods of complete or partial interruptions in breathing during sleep. A sensor is placed in or near the nostril and outside the mouth. In some cases, an additional cannula, or slender tube, is positioned near the nose to measure the amount of carbon dioxide in exhaled air. Two belts placed around the chest and abdomen measure breathing effort during sleep.

Oxygen saturation By measuring the oxygen level, the technologist can determine whether apneic events are producing significant drops in oxygen during sleep. To do this, a pulse oximeter probe is placed over the fingertip or ear lobe.

Body position The technologist records unusual body movement and sleep position by observing patients while they sleep and making a video recording of the overnight study. Video usage is becoming mainstream in sleep laboratories. Before the study begins, the technologist will indicate whether patients will be recorded and often obtains a written consent.

Snoring A snore microphone is taped to the lateral neck area.

How do I prepare for a sleep study?

The overnight sleep study should be tailored to fit your needs. To ensure that it will address your sleep concerns, your physician will be required to provide the sleep center with a recent medical history and physical examination prior to the test, as well as some details about the reason the test has been ordered (i.e., snoring, daytime sleepiness). Many centers will ask you to maintain a log of your sleep and wake times, including naps, for one to two weeks before testing. A sleep log not only provides insight to the technologist or physician who performs and reads (or "scores") your polysomnogram, it also can help you better understand your problem.

Additionally, patients often are requested to fill out questionnaires, like the Epworth Sleepiness Scale, prior to an overnight study. You might receive these questions in advance or be asked to answer them after you check into the sleep lab for your test. The questionnaires are a critical component of the overnight study, preparing sleep specialists with your sleep history information so they can better interpret the results.

If you drink coffee throughout the day, you should pare down to one cup in the morning in the weeks before your scheduled sleep study. Your study will not begin until your normal bedtime, so there is no reason to avoid caffeine completely, as long as you

Your sleep history should include information on:

- Snoring
- Witnessed apneas
- Choking or gasping during sleep
- Excessive daytime sleepiness
- Daytime fatigue
- Impaired concentration
- Difficulty falling sleep because of uncomfortable legs
- Recurrent awakenings from sleep
- Unusual behavior at night
- Excessive movements during sleep
- Medical history
- Past surgeries
- Medications, alcohol, and recreational drug use
- Weight change over time
- History of childhood sleep problems
- Family history of sleep disorders

eliminate it before midafternoon. Otherwise, go about your day as you normally would on the day of your sleep study. Just avoid nicotine, alcohol, and excessive exercise that might keep you awake longer than on a normal night.

Following these guidelines will ensure that your test is accurate and the best possible example of normal sleep for you:

- Avoid taking a nap on the day of the study.

- Avoid alcohol, excessive caffeine, sedatives, and stimulants for 24 hours before the study, unless you are otherwise directed by your doctor. In some cases, patients who use stimulants are advised to continue their usual medications.

- Eat your regular evening meal before you arrive at the sleep lab.

- On the day of the study, make sure your hair is free of oil, hair spray, and other products.

- Bring your medications and plan to take them as you normally would, unless a physician instructs otherwise.

- Bring comfortable sleepwear (pajamas are better than nightgowns), but avoid silk.

- Bring the completed sleep questionnaires if paperwork was given to you before the study.

- If you are using positive airway pressure therapy at home, bring your mask.

- Pack an overnight bag with toiletries, sleepwear, and your own pillow if you prefer.

What to Expect at the Sleep Lab

If sleeping soundly at home is a rarity, the thought of catching some z's in an unfamiliar place may seem impossible, especially if you know you will be recorded and observed during the process. However, most patients who check into a sleep lab for an overnight study sleep better than they expect. They are exhausted, and most of them find that sleeping with sensors doesn't disturb them once they are in an environment that fosters sound sleep.

Adding to the likelihood that you will fall asleep during your overnight stay in the sleep lab is the fact that sleep labs are designed to be comfortable. Your room will likely resemble a hotel suite. Sleep labs typically are outpatient facilities, which don't have the clinical feel of a hospital setting. That said, medical elements aren't entirely absent from the experience. The nightstand in your sleep lab room might contain controllers and devices necessary to conduct the polysomnogram.

Because of a burgeoning demand for overnight sleep studies, many medical centers have expanded their sleep labs to locations outside the medical center's campus. Some sleep centers are located inside hotels in nearby communities. The Cleveland Clinic is one such health system; its Sleep Disorders Center opened branches in Courtyard Marriott hotels. This has been a popular choice for patients.

Regardless of whether your sleep lab stay will take place in the hospital, in an outpatient clinic, or in an equipped hotel setting, you will be greeted and introduced to the process when you check in. Typically, you will be scheduled to arrive for your study in the evening, usually a couple of hours before your normal bedtime. You will be shown to your room and given time to settle in, change into your pajamas, and relax for a while. A technologist will hook up the equipment required for your study, which can take up to an hour or longer, depending on the nature of your test. He or she will place electrodes and sensors on your head, chin, and legs, and sensors around your nose, mouth, chest, and abdomen.

The electrodes and wires that connect to the various machines are fairly noninvasive. You will feel the eight sensors that have been placed on your head, the five spread on your chest and legs, and the tubes near your nostrils. You might even feel electric—wired for sleep, one might say. But as the technologist prepares you for the study, explaining each sensor and the purpose of the devices, you're likely to feel that the sensors are not restrictive and are critical to helping you sleep better in the future.

If you have any questions, ask them while the devices are being applied. The technologist can ease any concerns you have about the process and explain why each measurement device is important to compiling a complete picture of your sleep patterns. Be sure to mention any morning commitments. That way, you can arrange an appropriate wake-up call. Tests usually last until 6 or 6:30 A.M., and some patients are required to stay the entire next day for additional daytime testing. Because most sleep centers are located in outpatient settings manned by technologists (and not nurses), expect to bring and take your own medications during your stay. Notify the sleep center in advance if you or a loved one has special needs.

In most sleep centers, the sleep rooms are equipped with showers, so you can bathe, dress, and go directly to work if you're free to leave after the overnight recording.

For an inside look at a Cleveland Clinic's sleep laboratory, log on to *www.clevelandclinic.org/sleeptesting*.

Will I be able to go to work the next day?

If you are asked to participate in a multiple sleep latency test (MSLT—see section below), you will be required to stay at the lab throughout the day that follows your overnight stay, so you should plan on taking the day off.

I'm accustomed to sleeping with my spouse. can someone come with me?

Unless you require your spouse to assist you with functions like going to the restroom in the middle of the night, the sleep lab will be unable to accommodate a companion. The exception to that rule is if the patient is under 18 years old. In that case, the patient must be accompanied by a parent or guardian. Pullout sofas are often available in the sleep lab rooms for guests.

What's going on while I'm asleep?

While patients sleep, the technicians are busy in the control room. They watch video screens and log body position and unusual movements. They listen for snoring and abrupt breathing noises—a pulse oximeter probe measures your oxygen level, and the sensors placed near your nostrils and outside your mouth record your breathing patterns. If breathing problems are observed, your technologist might wake you up and ask you to try a continuous positive airway pressure device. The machine, which rests on a bedside table, forces air into a mask that fits around your nose and/or mouth and into your airway, keeping it open so you can breathe and sleep better.

During the night, technologists record many readings, including eye movement; sleep staging (when your body enters stages 1 through 3 and REM); leg movements; heart rate; respiration; oxygen; body position; and snoring (through a snore microphone). They take notes when they notice behavior in various sleep stages. For example, if they detect leg movements (common with periodic limb movement disorder in early sleep stages), they note this on a sleep chart.

Your study may also be videotaped; this is an important part of the study, because it allows technologists to review body positioning as it relates to sleep disturbances. If your study is scheduled for videotaping, your technologist will notify you of this in advance.

• • • Fast Fact • • •

Before the availability of digital recording, a one-night polysomnogram recording could consume between 1,000 and 1,500 feet of paper. Now virtually all laboratories record data using computer systems instead of paper-based machines.

• • •

What happens when I wake up?

When you wake up at the end of the study, the technologist stops the recording. You may be asked to fill out a questionnaire that might include the following questions:

1) How long did it take you to fall asleep last night?
2) How does this compare with the length of time it usually takes you to fall asleep?

3) How long do you feel you slept last night?
4) How many times did you wake up last night?

Reading the Polysomnogram

Polysomnograms are like sleep maps: The squiggly, wavy, and sometimes flat lines are produced by the recording device tell physicians whether a patient displays symptoms of a sleep disorder. These studies are critical to correct diagnosis and treatment.

But what do the lines mean?

Below is an EEG (brain wave) tracing of a patient who is awake. The lines are random and fast.

Wake

Below is a depiction of the slower waves of a patient who is drowsy.

Stage 1

This recording displays theta waves of stage 1 sleep. These waves are repetitive and look like small, jagged mountains. They are still relatively small. During this stage, the patient's eyes may rove back and forth, and the movement is recorded on an EOG tracing.

In the tracing that follows, you will notice a "sleep spindle" and "K complex," both of which are inherent in stage 2 sleep recordings.

Stage 2

K complex/sleep spindle

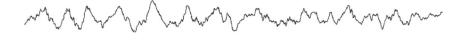

Stage 3 is characterized by high-voltage, slow delta waves. During a normal night's sleep, you spend most of your sleep time in stages 2 and 3.

Stage 3 Sleep

Approximately 90 minutes from sleep onset, REM sleep occurs. This type of sleep can happen three or more times a night. (It can occur less frequently if a patient displays problems

REM Sleep

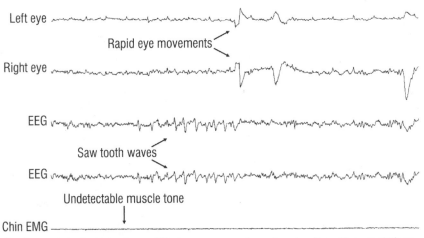

The figure at the bottom of page 20 shows a person's progression through normal sleep.

transitioning from one sleep stage to the next.) REM sleep is characterized by low-voltage waves that are random and fast with superimposed sawtooth-shaped waves.

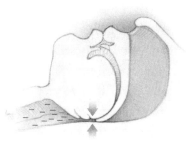

In cases of sleep apnea, video recordings are especially helpful because they allow a technologist to review a patient's sleep positions during the course of a night's sleep. For some patients, sleep apnea occurs only when the patient is sleeping on his or her back (because the position causes the tongue to flop backward, blocking the upper airway as shown in the figure below). The technologist will encourage a patient to sleep on his or her side and back, or supine, and in his or her usual sleep position (which might include sitting in a recliner). This allows the technologist to observe when the patient displays symptoms of sleep apnea.

Evaluating the Results

After an overnight sleep study, your doctor may refer you for a consultation with a sleep specialist to discuss the results, diagnosis, and treatment, as well as changes to sleep hygiene and lifestyle that will be critical to successful therapy.

How are sleep studies evaluated?

After the study is complete, the technologist scores the polysomnogram. It will take the technologist several hours to analyze the information and break it down into the following categories:

Time in Bed: Time from lights out to lights on, in minutes.

Total Sleep Time: Total time spent in stages 1 through 3 and REM, in minutes.

Sleep Latency: Time from lights out to the first appearance of sleep, in minutes.

REM Latency: Time from sleep onset to the first appearance of REM, in minutes.

Sleep Efficiency: Time in bed spent asleep, expressed as a percentage.

Sleep Stage Percentage: Time spent in each sleep stage divided by the total sleep time, expressed as a percentage.

Apnea/Hypopnea Indices: Number of apneic (total obstruction of the airway) or hypopneic (partial obstruction in breathing) events per sleep hour. More information about these conditions is available in chapter 5.

Arousal Index: Number of times per sleep hour an arousal from sleep occurs.

Oxygen Data: Number of times a patient experiences a significant reduction in oxygen, and the amount of sleep time spent with subnormal oxygen levels (expressed as a percentage).

PLMI Data: Number of periodic limb movements per sleep hour. Less than five per hour is normal for people under the age of 60. The cutoff is higher for mature adults, because PLMs increase with age.

PLMAI Data: Number of periodic limb movements per sleep hour that cause arousals. Many people have periodic limb movements, but physicians pay close attention when these movements trigger an arousal from sleep.

What is a sleep report?

After a technologist scores the study, a sleep specialist reviews it and prepares a report, based on the lab recording and your sleep history, for your physician. More than 2,000 variables are collected during an overnight sleep study, and the digitized programs in sleep recording systems crunch the numbers and allow doctors to sift through them to evaluate sleep disorders. For example, a doctor can find out whether you snore while you sleep on your back or on your right side. This may seem an insignificant detail, but it is important to know whether body position caused an apneic episode or whether disruptions in breathing occurred during a certain sleep stage. Tailored sleep study reports shed light on the intricacies of how we sleep.

• • • *Fast Fact* • • •

Because the environment of a sleep lab is new and different from the norm, patients often display minor aberrations in their usual sleep patterns. This is called first-night effect. These changes generally do not interfere with the interpretation of the study. However, in a minority of cases, a physician may request that a patient return to the lab for a second study to ensure accurate results.

• • •

Daytime Sleep Testing: the MSLT

In addition to the overnight polysomnogram, your physician might request that you stay at the sleep lab during the ensuing day to undergo a multiple sleep latency test, or MSLT. The MSLT is the gold-standard test used in the evaluation of daytime sleepiness. The test consists of five nap trials, performed at two-hour intervals, the day after an adequate night's sleep. The test indicates whether a patient has excessive daytime sleepiness and measures its severity. It is an important test for patients suspected of having narcolepsy, a disorder marked by uncontrollable sudden sleep attacks during active situations such as eating, talking, and even driving.

A technologist sets the stage for each nap by dimming lights and asking you to lie down and close your eyes. In between nap trials, you will have downtime to read, work on a laptop, or participate in another low-key activity. Many labs provide breakfast and lunch, but ask about this in advance.

Take Elizabeth, for example.

Elizabeth

Elizabeth's physician ordered a polysomnogram to get a better picture of how she spends her nights after she presented with symptoms of narcolepsy. After her overnight sleep study, during which she slept soundly, she was asked to stay for an MSLT.

When the technologist entered her room to prepare her for the first nap trial, Elizabeth was already sound asleep. Only seconds had passed since the technologist had turned off the light. Back in the control room, the technologist noticed that Elizabeth entered REM, abnormal behavior during a nap. When Elizabeth was awakened, she said she did not realize how soundly she had slept.

Nearly two hours later, it was time for the second nap trial. She fell asleep just as quickly.

The MSLT is based on the assumption that sleep is critical to function. When a patient is sleep-deprived or has a disorder in which wakefulness is impaired, the body will shut down—in other words, the patient will fall asleep quickly and deeply, much more so than is normal during a nap. Electrodes placed on the head to measure brain waves and eye movements indicate how deeply a patient sleeps during nap trials. Patients who fall asleep in five minutes or less display signs of severe, excessive daytime sleepiness. (Normally rested individuals generally do not fall asleep in less than ten minutes in this situation.)

In Elizabeth's case, the MSLT was critical to diagnosing her sleep disorder because it allowed the physician to discover how very little time it took Elizabeth to fall asleep, even after sleeping well at night. Since she was well rested, the results indicated that narcolepsy, as opposed to a nighttime sleep disturbance like sleep apnea, was responsible for her daytime sleepiness.

How do I prepare for daytime testing?

Daytime testing lasts for most of the day, so call the sleep lab in advance to find out detailed information about breakfast, lunch, and the approximate time the study will end. During the day, you should take prescribed medications as usual, unless you are otherwise instructed by your physician.

In order to prepare for daytime sleep trials, follow these steps:

- Bring reading materials or other activities to occupy free time between trials.
- Wear comfortable clothing.
- Avoid naps, smoking, or physical exertion prior to the test and in between nap trials.

What can I expect to happen during a daytime sleep study?

If you have spent the night at the sleep lab, a technologist will wake you in the morning and remove the respiratory, oxygen, and leg sensors. Only brain activity, eye movements, and muscle tone over the chin are measured during the MSLT, and these recordings are captured using the same electrodes applied the night before.

Most sleep laboratories will provide a light breakfast before the MSLT test begins. You will not be permitted to consume stimulants, alcohol, or caffeine (including your standard cup of morning coffee) unless otherwise directed by your physician.

No sooner than 90 minutes after you wake up, the technologist will return to the room to prepare you for your first nap. Lights are turned out and other distractions removed. Your sleep patterns are monitored during this time.

The amount you sleep during these nap trials fleshes out a physician's understanding of complaints of daytime sleepiness, fatigue, and disrupted sleep at night. The MSLT uncovers information that is critical to making an accurate sleep disorder diagnosis and designing a treatment plan.

Just over 50 years ago, the very first sleep recording consisted of a single EEG electrode placed on the head to detect different patterns of brain wave activity during the night. Sleep technology has come a long way in the years since then. Today, thousands of people are snoozing in sleep laboratories across the U.S. every night. But estimates are that this population represents only a small fraction of the total number of people with sleep disorders who would benefit from testing. If you suffer from unrefreshing sleep or daytime fatigue, talk with your doctor. He or she can review your sleep history and refer you to a sleep laboratory for testing or to a sleep specialist for further evaluation. Most insurance carriers will assess the need for a sleep study in advance and provide precertification. It is a good idea to contact your insurance company before the night of the test to find out if you are financially responsible for any portion of the laboratory charges.

And don't put it off! If you're like most patients, your sleep study will provide the critical answers your doctor needs to helping you get the sleep you need so that you too can enjoy restful nights and productive days.

Chapter 4

Diagnosis and Classification of Sleep Disorders

Sleeping is no mean art:
for its sake one must stay awake all day.

—**Nietzsche**

The body of knowledge about normal sleep and how the body should transition from one sleep stage to the next enables physicians to distinguish sleep disruptions that originate within the body from those initiated by outside influences. The tools we've previously discussed, such as an overnight sleep study, questionnaires, and sleep logs, can help your doctor diagnose your sleep disorder.

How many types of sleep disorders are there?

There are more than 80 sleep disorders, ranging from the mildly disruptive (such as adjustment insomnia—a transient type of insomnia caused by a stressor such as job loss or death in the family) to the

> The *International Classification of Sleep Disorders* (2nd ed.) was revised by the American Academy of Sleep Medicine in 2005. The manual describes the currently recognized sleep disorders based on available medical evidence. It serves as a sleep disorders reference for specialists.

extremely dangerous (narcolepsy—sleep attacks that occur without warning). Even the mildest sleep disorders may require an evaluation by a sleep specialist. As noted in Chapters 1 and 2, a lack of sleep can build up over time, creating a sleep deficit that deprives the body of time necessary to repair and rejuvenate itself. This situation, in turn, can lead to serious complications and health hazards, including high blood pressure, weight gain, anxiety and depression, academic under-achievement, poor work performance, and motor vehicle accidents.

Sleep disorders are classified in six major categories:

Insomnias These disorders present with the primary complaint of insomnia, defined by difficulty initiating or maintaining sleep, early morning awakening, or nonrestorative sleep despite adequate opportunity, resulting in daytime impairment.

Examples:

Adjustment insomnia (acute insomnia)

Psychophysiological insomnia

Inadequate sleep hygiene

Behavioral insomnia of childhood

Insomnia due to drug or substance, psychiatric disorder or medical condition

Sleep-related breathing disorders Sleep-related breathing disorders are characterized by disordered respiratory patterns in sleep.

A polysomnogram, along with a blood gas test or measure of lung capacity in some cases, is required to differentiate these.

Examples:

> Central sleep apnea syndromes
>
> Obstructive sleep apnea syndromes
>
> Sleep-related hypoventilation and/or hypoxemic syndromes
>
> Sleep-related hypoventilation and/or hypoxemia due to medical condition (pulmonary, neuromuscular or chest wall disorders)
>
> Other sleep-related breathing disorders

Hypersomnias of central origin Shared among these disorders is a primary complaint of daytime sleepiness or an inability to stay awake or alert during waking hours. Excluded are cases in which daytime sleepiness is primarily attributable to a sleep-related breathing disorder or a circadian rhythm disorder (see below).

Examples:

> Narcolepsy with/without cataplexy
>
> Recurrent hypersomnia
>
> > Kleine-Levin syndrome
> >
> > Menstrual-related hypersomnia
>
> Idiopathic hypersomnia with/without long sleep time
>
> Behaviorally induced insufficient sleep syndrome
>
> Hypersomnia due to drug or substance or medical condition

Circadian rhythm sleep disorders Circadian rhythm disorders are defined by the presence of a persistent or recurrent sleep disturbance caused by alterations of the internal body clock or misalignment between the body's internal rhythms and environmental factors.

Examples:

> Delayed sleep phase disorder
> Advanced sleep phase disorder
> Irregular sleep-wake rhythm
> Jet lag disorder
> Shift work disorder

Parasomnias These disorders are undesirable events or experiences that occur as one enters sleep, within sleep, or during arousals from sleep. In many cases, parasomnias are marked by complex, seemingly purposeful movements or behaviors and dreaming, often with emotional content.

Examples:

> Disorders of arousal (from NREM sleep)
>> Confusional arousals
>> Night terrors
>> Sleepwalking
> Parasomnias usually associated with REM sleep
>> REM behavior disorder
>> Nightmare disorder
> Other Parasomnias
>> Sleep enuresis
>> Exploding head syndrome
>> Sleep-related eating disorder
>> Parasomnia due to drug or substance or medical condition

Sleep-related movement disorders In contrast to the parasomnias, sleep-related movement disorders are characterized by relatively simple movements in sleep that nevertheless lead to sleep disruption or daytime sleepiness or fatigue.

Examples:

Restless legs syndrome

Periodic limb movement disorder

Leg cramps

Bruxism

Rhythmic movement disorder

Can sleep disorders be caused by other conditions?

Sleep disorders are also associated with psychiatric, behavioral, and physical conditions. Mood disorders, anxiety, depression, schizophrenia, and other psychotic and personality disorders often contribute to a person's inability to sleep. A physician must determine whether the individual does, in fact, present with a primary sleep disorder or whether the sleep problems are is a secondary symptom of a psychiatric or behavioral disorder.

Medical conditions that disrupt sleep include headaches, gastroesophageal reflux, sleep-related epilepsy and chest pains and pulmonary disorders such as chronic obstructive pulmonary disease.

Sleep affects our whole health, and the presence of a psychological or physical condition will have an effect on a patient's chances of getting a good night's sleep.

Chapter 5

Obstructive Sleep Apnea

Laugh and the world laughs with you; snore and you sleep alone.

—Anthony Burgess

Obstructive sleep apnea is characterized by repetitive episodes of complete (apnea) or partial (hypopnea) upper airway obstruction during sleep. Often the disorder's first signs are snoring, gasping for breath during sleep, and excessive daytime sleepiness. Take Dan, for example.

Dan

Dan, 43, drove to work early one morning, groggy as usual, his third cup of coffee propped on the dashboard. He lapsed into a daze, staring blankly at the road before him, ticks of yellow road stripe blurring in his side-view mirror. His speed gradually slowed to five miles less than the limit while his car crept closer to the berm.

Dan jolted awake when his head nodded. Exhaling anxiously, he realized that he had almost driven his car into the highway ditch. Although he sleeps about eight hours each night as a rule, he never feels refreshed in the morning, regardless of how much coffee he consumes.

Why am I so tired every day? He considered the last time he awoke not feeling exhausted in the morning. He pinpointed the feeling to about ten years ago.

Dan's wife also hasn't been too cheery in the morning. Karen is accustomed to his daily naps and lazy weekends, but his loud snoring during the night tests her patience in addition to depriving her of sleep. To interrupt Dan's snoring during the night, Karen elbows him in the gut and rolls him from his preferred supine sleeping position to his side. As a rule, she also pulls the covers over her head to muffle the sound. For his part, Dan is oblivious to the problem until Karen complains in the morning. On nights when Dan's snoring is particularly loud, Karen will retreat to the sofa in the living room.

Dan is a sturdy man with a thick neck and a large frame. His body mass index is 38 (normal is 18.5 to 24.9), and his family doctor has warned him to reduce the amount of fast food he consumes.

Three years ago, Dan was diagnosed with obstructive sleep apnea (OSA) and treated with continuous positive airway pressure (CPAP), which requires Dan to sleep while wearing a mask that delivers air into the nose and/or mouth. Dan wore the mask regularly for a year, but he didn't notice any benefit. He stopped using it until recently. Karen asked him to ease back into CPAP therapy, hoping it would reduce his labored breathing. It hasn't. They both know that Dan needs to seek treatment again.

Dan's Sleep Assessment

Sleep snapshot

Dan, an electrician, averages eight hours of sleep each night. More sleep generally does not make him feel more refreshed during the day. Typically he dozes off and on beginning at 6 P.M., shortly after dinner, while lounging in front of the television. Karen wakes him up to go to bed a few hours later.

Dan is aware that he is roused out of sleep two times during each night. He suffers from several symptoms—snoring, reflux symptoms, leg or arm jerks, the need to use the bathroom during the night—each of which might be responsible for waking Dan. After observing her husband tossing and turning, his body jolting and snoring throughout the night, Karen suspects that Dan awakens much more frequently each night. Dan never has a problem falling back asleep after his sleep is interrupted.

Dan wakes up every morning at 5 and arrives at work no later than 7:30. He often has a headache in the morning. He generally finishes his last electrical job at 3:30 P.M. Last year during his annual performance evaluation, his supervisor noted that Dan was "losing his edge" and not quite as efficient as he had been in the past. Dan recalls that on at least one occasion, he received an electrical shock when he started to nod off in the middle of a wiring job.

Excessive daytime sleepiness

Despite the hours Dan clocks in bed each night, he rarely feels rested when he wakes in the morning. To compensate for his fatigue, he usually sneaks in two catnaps during his breaks at work. On Saturdays, he sometimes picks up overtime shifts, but if he has free time and is not scheduled to work, Dan will sleep the whole weekend.

Dan has lived with excessive daytime sleepiness for more than ten years, and like many patients who report this condition, he has grown accustomed to fatigue and learned to compensate or write it off as "no big deal." But when a wake-up call occurs in an automobile, the sleepiness requires medical attention. Dan has never received a moving violation, but he's come close to having an accident several times.

Medical and family history

After his overnight sleep study three years ago, Dan was diagnosed with OSA and treated with CPAP. He says this therapy has not helped him. His new physician could not locate documentation of the prior evaluations or polysomnogram results.

Sleep-related breathing disorders Dan has never had nose or throat surgery and recalls no history of facial trauma. But his snoring has worsened over the past six years. During the same time, he's packed on more than 30 pounds. His snoring is especially bad when he falls asleep on his back. Most of the time, snoring has no serious side effects other than being an annoyance, but Dan also notes that he sometimes stops breathing or gasps for air during sleep.

Snoring is the sound that tissues in the nose and throat area make when the airway is not completely open. It is often the first indication of obstructive sleep apnea, and the physician immediately linked Dan's habit to his previous OSA diagnosis.

Physical examination Dan shows no sign of overbite or enlarged tonsils, both of which can be indications of OSA. His nasal airway is adequate, but the physician noticed that his mouth is characterized by a very low-lying soft palate. Dan's examination also revealed excessive tissue on his lateral pharyngeal wall, or pharynx area. Dan's neck circumference measures 18 inches, and patients with larger-sized collars are more susceptible to OSA (additional tissue can crowd the upper airway). His heart rate, blood pressure, and respiratory rate (the number of breaths per minute) are normal.

The physician was most concerned about Dan's neck size and upper airway structure, two physical traits typical of patients with OSA.

The diagnosis

The physician referred Dan to the sleep laboratory where another overnight sleep study confirmed the previous diagnosis of OSA. During the study, Dan stopped breathing 42 times per hour (that's an apnea-hypopnea index of 42), and he spent about 25 percent of his sleep time with subnormal oxygen levels. The physician ordered an urgent polysomnogram with CPAP titration (a polysomnogram performed with CPAP to identify the pressure setting that normalizes breathing). His home CPAP machine hadn't been checked or adjusted since he'd initially received it. If Dan's daytime sleepiness did not improve with this treatment, he would require further evaluation.

The physician asked Dan to discuss medical leave with his employer. She ordered him to refrain from driving, operating heavy machinery or dangerous equipment, and to avoid heights until his daytime sleepiness improved.

Further, the physician discussed treatment options with Dan, including general measures like avoiding alcohol before bed, losing weight, not sleeping on his back, and having surgery to correct physical obstructions in the airway passage.

All about Obstructive Sleep Apnea

Who gets obstructive sleep apnea?

The typical OSA patient looks a lot like Dan: a middle-aged, overweight male with a large neck, a longtime snoring habit, and a tendency to lag during the day. But this is not the only demographic that suffers from OSA.

An estimated 3 million men and 1.5 million women in the United States show symptoms of OSA. And despite the 2:1 ratio of men to women who present with the disorder, the gender gap closes in later years when women are more susceptible due to hormonal changes. Obstructive sleep apnea syndrome (OSAS), defined as at least five episodes of apnea or hypopnea per hour of sleep along with excessive daytime sleepiness, affects 4 percent of men and 2 percent of women. When using the definition of five episodes of apnea (total obstruction of airway) or hypopnea (partial obstruction of airway) per sleep hour, 24 percent of men and 9 percent of women meet the criteria. As both men and women age, OSA symptoms are more prevalent, and all overweight individuals are at risk.

More physicians are diagnosing patients with OSA, recognizing the disorder's morbidity in association with other serious medical problems, such as cardiovascular disease, hypertension, and stroke. Many of these problems also are linked to obesity. Most patients who have OSA are overweight and display weight gain prior to diagnosis.

How do I know if I have obstructive sleep apnea?

Obstructive sleep apnea is one of the most common sleep disorders, with nearly 25 percent of men and 10 percent of women who are diagnosed with a sleep disorder suffering from some degree of apnea. Often, bed partners are the first to detect early signs of OSA. Habitual snoring usually escalates in intensity before a patient is diagnosed with OSA. Many of those affected have no sleep complaints and feel refreshed when they wake up in the morning.

Although up to 30 percent of adults snore, those who present with OSA exhibit a loud, disruptive snoring pattern. Loud snores are followed by silence when a patient stops breathing, followed by a gasp for air—snore, silence, gasp. An OSA patient will repeat this cycle of apneic episodes, or periods when the patient's breathing stops and restarts, throughout the night.

Just as OSA patients generally do not realize the extent of their snoring, they also tend to overlook their daytime sleepiness. As sleep deprivation becomes a cultural norm, exhausted individuals tend to downplay sleepiness, even when physicians question their level of alertness during the day.

The symptoms that indicate obstructive sleep apnea include:

- Sudden awakenings following apneic episodes with a sensation of gasping, choking, or holding breath
- Daytime sleepiness, unintentional sleep episodes, unrefreshing sleep, fatigue, and rarely, insomnia
- Night sweats
- Morning dry mouth or sore throat from excessive snoring and respiratory stress
- Intellectual impairment, such as trouble concentrating, forgetfulness, or irritability
- Impotence
- Morning headaches

Certain physical traits and clinical features are characteristic of obstructive sleep apnea, including:

- Large neck circumference
- History of habitual snoring
- High body mass index or excessive weight
- Structurally abnormal or crowded airway passages, including a number of physical blockages such as nasal obstruction, a small jaw, a large tongue, a low-hanging soft palate, a large uvula, an overbite, or enlarged tonsils
- Hypertension (high blood pressure)

Symptoms in children are more subtle, but physicians commonly notice enlarged tonsils and adenoids. Surgery to remove tonsils is often helpful to alleviate the symptoms of children with OSA.

Another sign of OSA in children is sluggishness and poor performance in school. Daytime sleepiness often is misinterpreted as laziness in the classroom.

Signs that a child might have obstructive sleep apnea include:

- Daytime mouth breathing and swallowing difficulty

- Inward movement of the rib cage when breathing in

- Unusual sleeping positions (such as sleeping on hands and knees or with the neck hyperextended)

- Agitated arousals

- Excessive sweating at night

- Adenoidal face: dull expression, a bloated look, and swollen eyes

- Excessive daytime sleepiness

- Developmental delay, learning difficulties, decreased school performance, and behavioral disorders. *(There is a link between childhood diagnoses of attention deficit disorder or attention deficit-hyperactivity disorder and OSA; up to 25 percent of children with ADD or ADHD may also have OSA.)*

- Morning headaches

- Growth delay

- Frequent bed-wetting

What causes obstructive sleep apnea?

Sleep can be a potentially dangerous time for a person with OSA. During sleep, the muscles relax, including the muscles in the throat. A partial collapse of airway muscles causes snoring, but a complete collapse is an apnea, or respiratory stop. *Apnea* comes from the Greek word meaning "without wind." In patients with OSA, the

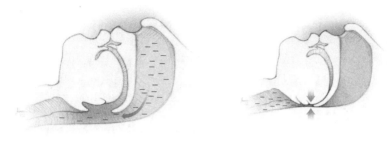

Normal airflow   *Restricted airflow*

throat muscles relax, narrow the breathing passages, and eventually collapse. The blockage causes apneic episodes—the snore, silence, gasp pattern familiar to bed partners of OSA sleepers.

Occasional apneas are normal, particularly in mature adults. But when apneas are repetitive and cause arousals, drops in a person's oxygen level, or changes in heart rate, they can contribute to more serious health problems.

OSA: The Polysomnogram

During an overnight sleep study, a patient's nasal and oral airflow are monitored through sensors placed in or near the nostrils and around the mouth. Two belts placed around the abdomen and rib cage measure breathing effort and are used to differentiate obstructive sleep apnea from a rarer condition known as central sleep apnea. An oximeter probe placed on the fingertip provides a measure of oxygen levels, a surrogate for the level of oxygen in the blood. Many times, apneas cause repetitive drops in oxygen that deprive the brain and heart of this vital nutrient. A snore microphone is taped on the side of the neck to measure the intensity of snoring and correlate it with breathing patterns.

During an apneic episode, airflow through the nose and mouth stops, often causing an arousal and/or a change in heart rate. The heart typically will slow (*bradycardia*) during the apnea and speed up (*tachycardia*) at the time of arousal. This is called a *bradytachy response.*

Coming Soon to a Home Near You

In 2008, the government agency that regulates Medicare and Medicaid approved coverage for CPAP therapy for OSA based on a diagnosis made during in-home testing. In the past, CPAP coverage was provided only to patients who were diagnosed by a PSG performed in an accredited sleep laboratory. In the coming years, it is expected that most labs will offer this option to some of their patients.

If you have medical problems that affect your heart or lungs or symptoms of other sleep disorders, you should seek immediate medical attention. In-home diagnosis is not for you. Portable monitoring devices that are used in the home should be used only to diagnose patients whom doctors deem to have a moderate to high likelihood of having OSA. They should not be used in cases of central sleep apnea, periodic limb movement disorder, insomnia, parasomnia, circadian rhythm disorder, or narcolepsy. In addition, in-home testing should be restricted to patients who have no other medical conditions that could interfere with the monitoring, such as heart failure or COPD. Portable monitoring devices are not recommended for diagnosing children and should be used with caution in seniors, who generally tend to have more medical problems.

The arousal is a reset button of sorts. After waking momentarily, patients catch their breath and fall back asleep. Most patients do not recognize these arousals. For example, Dan said he woke up only two times during the night. But his polysomnogram indicated that he was aroused from apneic episodes 42 times each hour.

Technologists look for breathing stops (apneic episodes) and episodes of significant breathing reduction (hypopneic episodes) that last at least 10 seconds in duration; most episodes last from 20 to 40 seconds, and some as long as between 60 and 90 seconds, though respiratory stops of this duration are rare. Episodes generally occur during NREM sleep stages 1 and 2, and they are more prevalent during REM. (Some patients experience these events only during REM sleep.) The human body can in fact go much longer without oxygen—about 3 to 4 minutes—before brain cells start to die. While patients with sleep apnea may have hundreds of apneas and hypopneas per night, these episodes are almost always associated with brief drops in oxygen that recover to normal in between events.

Obstructive Apnea

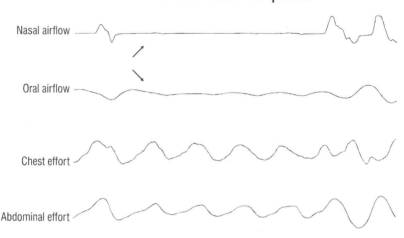

Arrows indicate an obstruction of airflow in the back of the throat preventing normal breathing in sleep.

How to Get a Good Night's Sleep

Treatment of OSA depends on the severity of the condition. A physician might suggest general measures (such as abstaining from alcohol before bed, altering sleep position, losing weight) and/or therapeutic treatment. The latter includes positive airway pressure (PAP) therapy, oral appliances that help open the airway, and/or surgery to correct physical abnormalities of the upper airway that prevent normal nocturnal breathing. More often today, bariatric surgery is considered to relieve the symptoms of morbidly obese patients. Stimulants are used to treat residual daytime sleepiness in some cases.

No one formula works for everyone, and physicians often employ a combination of approaches to combat OSA. The key is to discuss treatment goals with your physician. Patients whose chief complaint is severe daytime sleepiness are not prime candidates for upper airway surgery, which will usually cure snoring but may not make you feel more awake during the day. Some patients adjust well to PAP therapy, while others cannot tolerate the machine. This is why education and a thorough assessment are critical precursors to any treatment plan.

General measures

- Weight loss: Weight gain can produce excess tissue in the neck region, which contributes to airway collapse. Even moderate weight loss can improve breathing during sleep.

- Avoiding alcohol and central nervous system depressants before bed: These agents relax muscle tone, including in the nasal and throat passages.

- Sleeping position: Some patients exhibit OSA only when they sleep on their backs. In this position, tissue is more likely to fall back into the throat and prevent normal breathing. A side sleeping position is known to reduce apneic episodes. (To prevent sleeping on their backs, some OSA patients sleep in a tight-fitting shirt with a tennis ball lodged in the back; others position a pillow or maternity wedge behind them to prevent themselves from rolling over.)

- Nasal congestion: People with sinus problems or frequent nasal congestion are more likely to experience OSA. In some cases, medication can reduce snoring and open the airway for better nighttime breathing. Nasal strips also can reduce snoring. (Keep in mind, however, that these treatments help breathing but do not reverse OSA.)

Positive airway pressure therapy

There are several types of positive airway pressure (PAP) therapy the most common of which are: continuous (CPAP), bi-level (bi-PAP), and automatic (APAP). Each delivers air from a machine through a mask, which is technically known as an interface, and into a patient's airway. The airflow prevents nasal and throat passages from collapsing during sleep, thereby reducing apneic episodes. How air pressure is delivered depends on the type of machine.

Personalizing PAP therapy to fit an individual's specific treatment needs is critical to the therapy's success. This is why a consultation with a physician and an educational session prior to a patient using a machine are so important. A professional can assist you in choosing the correct mask and brief you on what to expect with the treatment.

Positive airway pressure therapy is a long-term solution for OSA, but some patients who do not allow time (up to two months) to adjust to the therapy abort the treatment before they can experience its benefits. Communication with a physician is especially important during the training wheel stages of PAP therapy. Tell your doctor if air pressure is too strong, if the mask chafes your skin, or if the machine noise bothers a bed partner (most of today's machines purr quietly and are not disruptive to sleep once patients and bed partners grow accustomed to the white noise). There is a wide assortment of PAP equipment on the market.

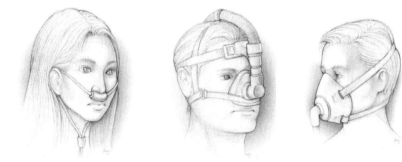

PAP masks come in a variety of styles and sizes.

Proper titration is necessary for CPAP treatment. A CPAP titration study is an overnight sleep study, similar to the polysomnogram, during which sleep is recorded using the same electrodes and sensors but with the addition of PAP. During this process, a sleep lab technologist will explain CPAP therapy and fit the patient with a comfortable mask or nasal cushions. The technologist monitors breathing and sleep quality during the night, and increases or decreases settings to determine which air pressure setting is best.

Positive airway pressure treatment is effective for about 90 percent of patients who use machines most of the time, but education and titration to determine appropriate air pressure are critical to the likelihood of successful outcome. When Dan was first diagnosed with OSA, he did not have a CPAP titration during the course of treatment. Therefore, his CPAP machine was probably not set at the appropriate pressure to abolish apnea episodes—and worse, he found the treatment uncomfortable. This explains why he felt the treatment was ineffective.

Common complaints among patients who use CPAP therapy include dry mouth, a leaking mask, sore or red eyes, nasal congestion, and skin irritation from the mask. Consultation with a physician may prevent these aggravations or minimize them so the treatment is tolerable. Continuous positive airway pressure can effectively control OSA as long as a patient commits to using it on a nightly basis.

Oral appliances

If you have mild OSA, you might benefit from a device that advances the tongue or jaw forward to open the airway. Although this method is usually not sufficient to treat severe OSA, patients who cannot tolerate CPAP therapy might respond to this alternative. However, not everyone is a good candidate for this approach. For example, patients without teeth (edentulous) and those with severe TMJ (temporomandibular junction) or periodontal disease cannot use most appliances. A sleep specialist and a dentist or prosthodontist with expertise in oral appliances for this purpose should jointly determine whether this treatment is best for you.

When it comes to dental appliances, one size doesn't fit all. That's why many specialists recommend adjustable devices that can be tailored to the anatomic needs of the individual. To alter the fit, the OSA patient periodically adjusts a crank on the device. This expands the device and gradually advances the jaw forward.

Surgery

In recent years, the list of upper airway surgical procedures to treat snoring and sleep apnea has increased drastically. This includes minimally invasive approaches performed by an otolaryngologist (ear, nose, and throat specialist) in the office or same-day surgery. Among the most commonly performed procedures are:

- Somnoplasty: In this procedure, radio waves are used to shrink tissue in the airway. The soft palate, tongue, or throat is pierced with an electrode that is connected to a radio frequency generator, and the inner tissue is heated, causing it to shrink.

- Laser-assisted uvuloplasty: A surgical procedure to remove the uvula and surrounding tissue to open the airway behind the palate. This procedure has been used to relieve snoring.

- Tonsillectomy: The most effective treatment for snoring and sleep apnea in younger individuals, the procedure is sometimes used to treat adult snorers and apnea patients, too.

- Nasal septoplasty and turbinate reduction: These procedures straighten the nasal septum and reduce tissue inside the nose, improving nasal breathing and eliminating snoring or improving tolerance to PAP.

- Uvulopalatopharyngoplasty (UPPP or U- Triple P): The *uvulo* refers to the uvula, the fleshy piece of tissue that hangs in the back of your throat, *palato* refers to the palate, and *pharyngoplasty* means plastic surgery of the pharynx. The pharynx is the part of the throat that begins behind the nose and extends to the voice box and esophagus, and it serves as a channel to conduct both air and food. During the procedure, the uvula is removed along with excess tissue. This surgery is usually considered for patients who cannot tolerate PAP, but it has mixed results and cures sleep apnea in only a minority of cases.

In some cases, procedures are combined to achieve a better result.

Also available are more extensive procedures designed to eliminate obstruction in the airway. One of these is mandibular myotomy (the mandible is the lower jaw bone, and a myotomy is a surgical division of a muscle) with genioglossus (chin and tongue) advancement. This approach involves cutting a rectangular piece of bone in the front part of the jaw where the tongue muscles attach, pulling it and rotating it outward, and then reattaching it, which in effect pulls the tongue forward, eliminating the sleep-related obstruction. This procedure is a major undertaking and should be performed only by skilled, experienced surgeons. Oftentimes, an otolaryngologist and maxillofacial surgeon team up to perform this procedure.

Tracheostomy is rarely performed today, but it is perhaps the most effective way to resolve life-threatening cases of OSA. This procedure involves creating a hole, or stoma, in the neck. A tube is inserted in the hole to bypass the obstruction in the nose or throat.

Before recommending any type of surgery, a sleep specialist and surgeon must determine whether the patient's goal is realistic. If a patient's complaint is limited to snoring, breaking and reforming the jaw is an extreme measure to stop the sound. By contrast, somnoplasty—a much less invasive solution—cures snoring in nearly 100 percent of cases. However, if the patient weighs 300 pounds, somnoplasty won't stop OSA. During the course of a patient's evaluation, a physician will explain whether a procedure is necessary, conduct a risk assessment, and determine whether the surgery's results will meet the patient's desired outcome.

Dan's Outcome

After the sleep study, a specialist evaluated Dan and conducted an educational session about OSA. Dan was fitted with a new mask and headgear (the straps and other essentials needed to keep the CPAP device securely in place during sleep). Dan was surprised at how large a selection of masks was available to him. During his first course of therapy, he received his machine but little instruction provided and no choice of mask.

Dan learned how to maintain the equipment so it was clean and minimized the chance of bacteria buildup. His machine was equipped with a heated humidifier, and Dan was given a chinstrap to keep his mouth closed while he slept at night so the air forced through the mask would not escape through his mouth. Dan and Karen were counseled on the importance of using CPAP *all night, every night* to maximize its effect. Given that Dan's apnea is in the severe range, he is at risk for high blood pressure, heart attack, stroke, and diabetes should he fail to take this seriously.

Dan used the equipment nightly for the first few weeks. But after his follow-up visit a few weeks later, Dan started taking an occasional night off from the CPAP machine. Both he and Karen suffered the consequences: Karen couldn't sleep those nights, and Dan had trouble staying awake the following days. He quickly learned that spending a few minutes before bed each night to secure the mask was a healthy choice for both of them.

Within the first year of treatment, Dan was able to resume an exercise program, using the time he had spent napping, and he eventually lost some weight. He returns every year to the sleep clinic for reevaluation.

Chapter 6

Narcolepsy

Even where sleep is concerned, too much is a bad thing.
—Homer

N arcolepsy's hallmark is excessive daytime sleepiness characterized by repeated episodes of "naps" or lapses into sleep. For example, consider Felicia.

Felicia

Falling asleep is never a problem for Felicia, who conks out moments after her head hits the pillow. Even if one of her typical bouts of acid reflux burns in her chest, she is usually able to roll over to her left side and easily slip back into a deep sleep that lasts until the alarm sounds at 5:30 A.M. Felicia likes to get to the office before the rest of her staff, and her workload as executive vice president of a marketing firm demands extra hours in the office.

Despite work stress, Felicia never has a problem falling asleep. But strangely, she never feels rested. She assumes this is because of her early wake-up time.

Lately, Felicia's days have been punctuated by what she calls "slips," when her mind and body check out. For example, sometimes while driving to work, she will hit a speed bump that jerks her out of a daze. She admits that her husband, Reynold, nudges her during car trips—even short ones—so she won't daydream or have a head bob while she's at the wheel. He knows she works hard during the day, so he never questions her catnaps before dinner or during her lazy Sundays. She may sleep on the couch for hours at a time if she doesn't have to run errands.

After prodding from Reynold, Felicia visited a doctor to discuss her fatigue and sluggishness. During a sleep interview, the doctor learned that she slept about nine hours each night, going to bed between 8:30 and 9 on work nights. The specialist asked Felicia about her sleep hygiene, daytime sleepiness, breathing, movements, and any habits she noticed during sleep. Felicia's weekdays follow a predictable routine. She fuels up with a morning cup of coffee at home and then stops at the coffee shop near her office for a refill, arriving at work around 7 A.M. She takes several coffee breaks throughout the morning.

By the time Felicia gets home at 5:30 P.M., she's exhausted. She and Reynold fix dinner and share a cup of tea after their meal. Felicia usually dozes off in her chair and eventually retires to the bedroom.

Felicia's Sleep Assessment

Sleep snapshot

Felicia practices good sleep hygiene. She doesn't watch television, eat, or read in bed. She reports falling asleep immediately, waking up only to go to the bathroom or because of a sudden leg jerk or shortness of breath. She experiences reflux symptoms, but her heartburn has subsided since she quit smoking. She stopped having her nightly glass of red wine some years ago, as it usually made her feel even sleepier during the next day.

Excessive daytime sleepiness

Felicia admits that she never feels refreshed in the morning, no matter how long she has slept during the preceding night. She sneaks in several catnaps a day and says she would sleep all day if she could. Drowsy driving is a concern. Felicia has never had a car accident or received a moving violation, but she is able to fall asleep during a stoplight and will roll down windows to stay awake, even during short drives.

To evaluate her daytime sleepiness, Felicia took the Epworth Sleepiness Scale. When the physician evaluated her test, Felicia scored a 19, suggesting severe daytime sleepiness. Scores of 10 and higher are abnormal.

Following are some questions your physician might ask you to determine the cause and severity of excessive daytime sleepiness:

1. Do you feel sleepy no matter how much sleep you get?

2. Do you fall asleep in inappropriate situations or find yourself fighting to stay awake while driving or in meetings, even after a full night's sleep?

3. Do you experience spells of muscle weakness when you are happy, sad, or angry?

4. Do you dream during short naps?

5. Do your family or friends describe situations in which your sleepiness was unusual or memorable? (Many narcoleptics were the joke of their family on trips and family events.)

6. Do you use caffeine excessively to stay awake (including pills and beverages with high quantities of caffeine)?

7. Do you find yourself in places without knowing how you got there or have you lost time in the middle of a task?

8. Do you snore or wake up gasping for air?

9. During the night, do you experience uncomfortable sensations in your legs that are relieved by stretching or walking?

10. Do you sleep much longer on weekends than during the week?

If you answered *yes* to the first seven questions, you may have narcolepsy.

If you snore regularly, you should be evaluated for sleep apnea. A diagnosis of both narcolepsy and sleep apnea is possible if symptoms of both are evident through your polysomnogram and sleep questionnaires.

Restless legs syndrome is a common disorder in which unusual leg sensations interfere with one's ability to fall asleep or stay asleep. (See chapter 7 for more information on restless legs syndrome.)

Finally, if you sleep much later on weekends than on weekdays, your body may be simply refueling its stores from insufficient sleep during the week. Insufficient sleep syndrome, rampant in modern society, is the most common cause of daytime sleepiness.

Medical and family history

In addition to reflux symptoms, Felicia has asthma. Her father has diabetes. Her grandmother had throat cancer. She says that sleep disorders do not run in her family, but she notes that her father snored and her mother often took naps during the day. Felicia had a great-aunt who slept excessively and told tales at family gatherings about her vivid dreams.

The risk of developing narcolepsy is 1 to 2 percent in first-degree relatives of narcoleptics. Narcoleptics also have a higher risk of obesity and Type 2 diabetes mellitus, which may relate to dysfunction in the hypocretin-secreting cells of the hypothalamus.

Felicia's aunt displayed characteristics of narcolepsy, though she was never formally diagnosed with the disorder. Her father's history of diabetes puts Felicia at risk for this disease as well.

Insomnia

Felicia does not display signs of insomnia and says she has not experienced recent changes in life events. She says her bedroom is comfortable, and sleep onset is immediate. After learning about Felicia's sleep habits earlier, the doctor ruled out insomnia.

Narcolepsy

Felicia's high ESS score and complaints of daytime sleepiness struck a chord with the physician. When asked whether she ever felt weak in her legs, arms, or jaw when she felt strong emotions, Felicia told a story that led to her diagnosis.

"Have you ever lost control over your body when you were laughing at a joke or were angry?" the physician asked Felicia.

"Like when my dog pees on the carpet?"

"What happens then?" asked the doctor.

"I get so mad that I can't talk or move."

Felicia told the doctor that she has had the experience of reaching out to scold the dog, losing muscle control in her legs, and dropping to her knees.

Perfect cataplexy, the doctor thought to herself.

Cataplexy is an abrupt decrease in or loss of muscle tone, and it is frequently elicited by laughter, anger, or surprise. It occurs in more than two-thirds of patients with narcolepsy. Typically during a cataplectic episode, the jaw sags, head falls forward, arms drop to the side, and the knees unlock or buckle. Severity ranges from complete paralysis to limited muscle loss to a quick sensation of weakness.

Physicians sometimes overlook short cataplectic attacks, like those described by Felicia, because they do not occur during sleep studies and they do not resemble full-blown attacks.

Felicia's doctor performed an examination and found no evidence of obstruction in the nose or throat area and normal breathing and heart sounds. Neurologically, Felicia's muscle strength was normal and when the doctor tapped on Felicia's arms and legs with a hammer, her reflexes were normal throughout. She was able to walk steadily heal-to-toe.

The diagnosis

In addition to her complaints about daytime sleepiness, Felicia also occasionally displays sleep paralysis. Common in patients with narcolepsy, this behavior occurs when the brain is awake, but the body remains in the motionless state characteristic of REM. During one of these episodes a patient's mind is saying, "Move!" But his or her body resists the command. This conflict is scary and confusing for patients.

Considering Felicia's excessive daytime sleepiness, cataplectic behavior, reports of occasional sleep paralysis, and excessive use of caffeine, the doctor determined that she might have a disorder known as narcolepsy with cataplexy. She ordered Felicia not to drive until after an overnight sleep study and multiple sleep latency test.

During the overnight study, people with narcolepsy also may present with symptoms of sleep apnea or other disorders. More often, however, narcoleptics display disruptions in normal sleep patterns with frequent awakenings not explained by apnea. During an MSLT, the patient takes five nap trials at two-hour intervals, beginning 90 minutes to three hours after the morning awakening. Narcoleptics generally fall asleep at every opportunity, often in less than five minutes, while normal people stay awake the entire time or fall asleep no sooner than ten minutes after each trial starts. In addition, most people with narcolepsy fall quickly into REM sleep, known as sleep-onset REM periods. Felicia's MSLT and polysomnogram demonstrated all these features, with a mean sleep latency (the average time to fall asleep across five nap trials) of 4.6 minutes. Sleep-onset REM periods occurred during two of the five trials.

After reviewing results from the polysomnogram and MSLT, the doctor diagnosed Felicia with narcolepsy and prescribed a stimulant.

All about Narcolepsy

Who gets narcolepsy?

Anyone can get narcolepsy, but the disorder does seem to have a genetic component. Excessive daytime sleepiness—the main symptom of narcolepsy—generally surfaces in the early teens and twenties. Narcolepsy is less likely in older adults, but it can begin at any age.

Many narcoleptics learn to cope with their disease. In fact, most have learned how to work, play, and live with sleepiness because they grew up tired. Narcolepsy can range in severity, and some patients regard their sleepiness as merely an inconvenient nuisance that forces them to doze during conversations or in situations that do not require active participation. On the other hand, other patients experience narcolepsy as is a life-threatening illness, especially in cases where patients fall asleep while operating automobiles or heavy machinery. These patients display sudden, uncontrollable sleep attacks during active situations in which normal sleep never occurs.

How do I know if I have narcolepsy?

A common complaint of narcoleptics is that a 20-minute nap is refreshing, but a couple of hours later, they are sleepy again. Bosses often view narcoleptics (unfairly) as lazy and unmotivated, especially if they are aware of the narcoleptic's frequent naps and observe extreme sleepiness on the job. Relationships with spouses and family members also can suffer, because narcoleptics seem lethargic or uninterested. In truth, the problem is that the narcoleptic is exhausted beyond his or her control.

Many symptoms of narcolepsy are attributable to the abnormal tendency of patients to slip almost instantly from wakefulness into REM sleep. Symptoms include:

- Excessive daytime sleepiness (usually the first identified symptom)

- Recurrent daytime naps or lapses into sleep that occur almost daily for at least three months

- Disturbed sleep

- Automatic behavior: continuation of apparently normal behavior like taking a test or driving, without memory or awareness

- Pathological manifestations of REM sleep (such as cataplexy, sleep paralysis, and hypnagogic hallucinations)

Several other conditions may be associated with narcolepsy, creating separate diagnoses depending on the presentation of certain symptoms.

Cataplexy In this state, narcoleptics experience a sudden loss of muscle tone provoked by laughter, joking, surprise, or anger. During a cataplectic episode, consciousness remains clear, memory is not impaired, and respiration is intact, although the patient cannot speak or respond. Cataplexy usually lasts a few seconds to several minutes, and patients recover gradually over a few minutes. A patient can suffer from daytime sleepiness and present symptoms of narcolepsy but not experience cataplexy for up to 30 years. Cataplexy rarely precedes sleepiness. The frequency of attacks varies from a few in a lifetime to many per day. Some patients avoid emotional situations for fear of a cataplectic attack.

Sleep paralysis This is a transient inability to move or speak during the transition between sleep and wakefulness. Sleep paralysis is often paired with a sensation of inability to breathe, which frightens patients.

Most narcoleptics experience sleep paralysis; episodes usually resolve in a few minutes. They occur in 40 to 80 percent of narcoleptics.

Hypnagogic hallucinations These vivid perceptual experiences occur at sleep onset (or in the transition from sleep to wakefulness, in which case they are called hypnopompic hallucinations), generally with awareness of the presence of a person or thing. Often, hypnogogic hallucinations include abnormal perceptions of sight, sound, movements, and touch. Patients might describe hallucinations such as running from danger, flying through the air, or feeling as if someone or something is touching them. They are about as common as sleep paralysis in narcoleptics.

Low hypocretin levels Cells in the hypothalamus, deep in the brain, regulate wakefulness. These cells secrete a peptide called hypocretin. When researchers performed spinal taps to extract cerebrospinal fluid (CSF) of narcolepsy patients (as might be done to evaluate for meningitis), they discovered a deficiency in hypocretin. In recent years, such studies have sparked ideas that narcolepsy is a degenerative process that destroys hypocretin, which keeps a person awake. If true, this hypothesis would explain why narcoleptics fall asleep: they lack a substance in their brains that tells the body to stay awake. Low (CSF) hypocretin levels are seen in 90 percent of patients with narcolepsy and cataplexy, but almost never in healthy people or patients with daytime sleepiness that can be attributed to other disorders.

What is hypersomnia?

Felicia's symptoms clearly signified that she has narcolepsy with cataplexy. (Narcoleptic patients who do not have cataplexy may have more difficulty securing a diagnosis of their disorder.) Hypersomnia is the opposite of insomnia—hypersomniacs sleep a lot and still feel sleepy. Because our society does not always recognize serious sleepiness as a medical issue, many people who suffer from hypersomnia write it off as just being "really tired." While sleeping more is effective in reducing daytime sleepiness, patients with hypersomnia have an underlying disorder not helped by earlier bedtimes and more time allocated to sleep.

During an MSLT, hypersomniacs may display symptoms similar to those of narcoleptics, including low sleep latency and an occasional sleep-onset REM period. This is why keeping a sleep log prior to sleep lab testing is critical for a proper diagnosis. A sleep log will help your doctor rule out unusual sleep-wake cycles that might be causing hypersomnia. The log also demonstrates how much sleep is normal for you, so your doctor can compare your sleeping habits to overnight polysomnogram and MSLT results.

On the morning of the MSLT, you may be asked to supply a urine sample for a drug screen to rule out drug use as a cause of hypersomnia. Medications that suppress REM sleep, such as stimulants and antidepressants, should be discontinued before the study. In order to secure untainted results in the MSLT, a period of two weeks off such medications is recommended.

In most cases, the cause of narcolepsy is unknown and is presumably caused by low hypocretin levels in the central nervous system. Both genetic and environmental factors can predispose an individual to narcolepsy. The risk of a first-degree relative of a narcoleptic developing the disorder is at least ten times greater than the chances of anyone else in the population developing the disorder. Head injuries and viral illnesses before the onset of hypersomnia is found in some cases. Even rarer are cases of narcolepsy associated with brain disorders including multiple sclerosis, stroke, and brain tumors.

The Polysomnogram

A polysomnogram and MSLT of a narcolepsy patient will reveal one or more of the following symptoms:

- Sleep latency of less than ten minutes (time it takes to fall asleep).

- REM sleep latency of less than 20 minutes (sleep-onset REM period) on the polysomnogram.

- Increased amount of stage 1 sleep and frequent arousals and awakenings.

- A mean sleep latency on the MSLT of less than eight minutes, and usually less than five minutes, and two or more sleep-onset REM periods. However, up to 25 percent of narcoleptics may lack these findings.

How to Get a Good Night's Sleep

General measures

These general measures can lessen excessive sleepiness in narcoleptics:

- Take regular naps daily but limit them to about 20 minutes
- Limit use of alcohol
- Avoid central nervous system depressant medications, unless prescribed by your doctor
- Use caffeine in moderation to increase alertness
- Maintain regular sleep and wake-up times
- Avoid sleep deprivation

• • • *Fast Fact: When Sleepiness Strikes* • • •

Whether you have narcolepsy, sleep apnea, or intentionally stay up until the wee morning hours, here are some quick pick-me-ups when sleepiness sets in:

- Take a 20-minute nap
- Indulge in a shot of espresso or a chocolate bar, but do this in moderation

- Get up and get some exercise
- Turn down the thermostat: excessive heat induces slumber
- Turn on the lights: a well lit room will increase alertness

• • •

A Word on Caffeine

Found in coffee, teas, soft drinks, chocolate confections, and some over-the-counter and prescription medications, caffeine is the most commonly consumed drug in the world. Caffeine is a methylxanthine that blocks adenosine receptors in the brain, improving mental alertness and wakefulness. A typical 12-ounce cup of coffee contains 120–375 mg of caffeine. Caffeine is absorbed within 15–120 minutes and its effects last for a couple of hours. If ingested late in the day, it can cause insomnia. Excessive use can cause restlessness, agitation, tremors, palpitations, high blood pressure, increased urination, and rapid, shallow breathing.

A recent study performed by researchers at Walter Reed Army Institute of Research compared the effects of caffeine-containing chewing gum and placebo during a period of sleep deprivation. After 8 hours of sleep, subjects were asked to remain awake for the next 29 hours and complete computerized tests of attention, concentration, and motor speed. Not surprisingly, subjects given placebo made many more test errors than those given caffeine. The smallest number of errors occurred with highest doses of caffeine. Test performance was similar to baseline (before subjects had been sleep-deprived) when caffeine was administered at a dose of 200 mg every two hours—roughly the dose in an average cup of coffee. (See appendix 3 for caffeine contents of some popular beverages.)

In patients with narcolepsy and similar disorders, using caffeine at strategic times of the day can reduce the need for prescription medications.

Medications—narcolepsy The ideal wakefulness-promoting agent produces a maximally alert state without side effects or negative impact on one's ability to sleep when desired. There is a variety of available substances, although many are limited by tolerance and abuse potential. The FDA strictly regulates many of these compounds.

As with any stimulant, you should know that side effects are similar to those of being over-caffeinated: agitation, nervousness, and heart palpitations. Because tolerance develops over time with some agents, start with a low dose and very slowly work up to a larger dose. Never adjust the dose yourself as this can lead to life-threatening reactions.

Commonly prescribed medications used to treat excessive day-time sleepiness include:

Amphetamine (am-fet-a-meen), Dextroamphetamine (dec-troe-am-fet-a-meen), and Methamphetamine (meth-am-fet-a-meen)

Brand Names: *Adderall, Adderall XR, Dexedrine, Dexedrine SR,* Dextrostat, *Vyvanse, Desoxyn*

Amphetamine and related drugs such as dextroamphetamine and methamphetamine are a group of drugs that increase levels of the chemicals in the brain (dopamine, norepinephrine and sero-tonin) that sustain alertness and concentration. These drugs are also used illegally as recreational drugs and as performance enhancers. Dextroamphetamines have an increased affinity for dopamine receptors in the brain and are, therefore, more effective than amphetamine. The methylated form, known as methamphetamine, has increased central nervous system penetration, which renders it the most potent form in this class. These agents are associated with a variety of side effects, including loss of appetite, increased/distorted sensations, restlessness, headache, palpitations, diarrhea, blurred vision, uncontrollable movements or shaking, insomnia, and arrhythmias. Seizures and psychosis are rarely encountered. With prolonged use and/or high doses, tolerance can develop, therefore increasing the amount of the drug that is needed to maintain wakefulness.

Methylphenydate (meth-il-fen-i-date)

Brand Name: *Concerta, Metadate CD, Metadate ER, Methylin, Methylin ER, Ritalin, Ritalin LA, Ritalin-SR, Focalin (dexmethylphenidate), Focalin XR*

In use since the 1950s, methylphenidate is approved by the U.S. Food and Drug Administration for the treatment of both attention deficit hyperactivity disorder and narcolepsy. Researchers have found it effective in increasing alertness, and it is better tolerated than other drugs in the amphetamine class. Because methylphenidate also increases activity in other parts of the nervous system, untoward side effects are common. These include irritability, gastrointestinal problems, headache, nervousness, palpitations, high blood pressure, and disturbed nighttime sleep.

Modafinil (moe-daf-i-nill)

Brand Name: *Provigil*

The newest wakefulness-promoting drug on the block, modafinil is approved for the treatment of daytime sleepiness associated with narcolepsy, obstructive sleep apnea, and shift work sleep disorder (read more about this in chapter 11). Modafinil acts more selectively in the part of the brain called the hypothalamus, which regulates sleep and wakefulness functions. As a result, side effects tend to be mild and short-lived, typically limited to headache, nausea, and nervousness. For women taking oral contraceptives, an alternative form of contraception should be encouraged because this drug can reduce hormone concentrations, thereby leading to unexpected pregnancy. Although modafinil is less potent than the other drug classes, its low abuse potential and favorable side effect profile have made it a first-line treatment for patients who have not taken wakefulness-promoting medications in the past.

Please note: the use of wakefulness-promoting agents has been associated with high blood pressure and heart arrhythmias. If you are taking any of these medications, you should be closely monitored by your doctor.

Before beginning a regimen of any wakefulness-promoting drug, tell your doctor about any other pills you are taking, including prescription and over-the-counter medications, vitamins, minerals, herbal products, and drugs prescribed by other doctors. Do not start a new medication without telling your doctor.

These drugs may be habit-forming and should be used only by the person for whom the prescription was written. Keep the medication in a secure place that is out of the reach of children and individuals with drug or alcohol addiction problems. If you share living space with people you do not know well or may not be able to trust, consider storing the medication in a locked box or safe. I've found this storage strategy to be particularly useful for college students who live in dormitories.

Before using any wakefulness-promoting medication, tell your doctor if you are allergic to any drugs or

- if you have a history of heart problems, high blood pressure, blood vessel problems, or you have had a recent *heart attack*;

- if you have cirrhosis or other liver problems, epilepsy or seizures, an overactive thyroid, kidney disease or glaucoma;

- if you have a history of alcohol or other substance abuse;

- if you take *blood pressure medications*;

- if you have or any family member has a history of mental or mood problems (e.g., *bipolar disorder*, depression, psychosis), uncontrolled muscle movements (e.g., tics), Tourette's syndrome, or suicidal thoughts or attempts; and

- if you have a family history of sudden death or heart rhythm problems,

Also tell your doctor if you are pregnant, breast-feeding, or plan to become pregnant during treatment as many medications can cause harm to an unborn baby.

All wakefulness-promoting drugs affect the central nervous system. This can cause effects that may impair your thinking or reactions. Avoid dangerous activity, especially driving, until you know how this medication will affect your level of wakefulness.

Medications—cataplexy

During the 1970s and 1980s, cataplexy was treated primarily with tricyclic antidepressants (TCAs) such as protriptyline, clomipramine and imipramine. These drugs were (and remain) effective in ameliorating or eliminating cataplexy, sleep paralysis, and hypnagogic hallucinations, but they produce untoward effects such as dry mouth, blurred vision, and orthostatic hypotension (blood pressure drops while the patient is upright).

Newer selective serotonin reuptake inhibitors (SSRIs), such as fluoxetine, are as effective as the tricyclics but produce fewer side effects. Venlafaxine, a medication that increases both serotonin and norepinephrine in the brain, appears to be particularly effective in the treatment of cataplexy.

In 2002, the U.S. Food and Drug Administration approved Xyrem (sodium oxybate), the first drug specifically approved to treat cataplexy. Xyrem's history is recreational—it was abused as a date-rape drug, which explains why the substance is tightly controlled and available in the U.S. only through a single central pharmacy. The benefit of Xyrem is that it reduces cataplectic episodes by 85 percent while also reducing excessive daytime sleepiness. Xyrem also improves the fragmented sleep of narcoleptics.

The value of naps

Naps improve alertness and performance in sleep deprivation sufferers and people with narcolepsy and related disorders. Following are some useful facts about naps:

- Naps as short as 15 minutes in duration can significantly improve a person's ability to function at home, at work, and behind the wheel.

- Naps sustain performance, mood, and alertness longer than caffeine.

- Naps should last no longer than 2 hours to minimize sleep inertia (feelings of grogginess, hypovigilance, and impaired cognitive and behavioral performance that persist longer than few minutes after waking up suddenly from deep sleep).

- Napping before a night shift or before a long drive will reduce and delay feelings of sleepiness.

Felicia's Outcome

Felicia was diagnosed with narcolepsy with cataplexy and educated about the importance of maintaining strict bedtime and wake times, including on weekends. The physician warned her to avoid all drugs (including alcohol) that depress the central nervous system and contribute to daytime sleepiness. Many narcoleptics find that five-minute catnaps are extraordinarily effective, and Felicia was instructed to take at least two scheduled naps daily to ward off unscheduled sleep episodes.

Felicia's doctor took a few extra minutes to warn her about drowsy driving. Since the chances of falling asleep are very high when you drive drowsy, he told her to avoid this at all costs. Instead, he suggested the following:

- Take a 20-minute nap or drink a cup of coffee before getting behind the wheel.

- Find a ride, take a taxi, or use public transportation if you do not think you are alert enough to drive.

- Pull off the road to nap. Long monotonous driving, such as on the freeways, can make you sleepy, especially when you are sleep-deprived.

Lastly, Felicia's doctor pointed out the strategies that don't work, including turning up the radio, opening windows, chewing gum, or slapping/pinching oneself.

Following these simple measures, Felicia was prescribed the wakefulness-promoting medication Provigil (modafinil, 200 mg). She was directed to take the medication upon awakening to improve alertness. This initial dose had only a modest effect and was gradually increased to 600 mg per day. Excessive daytime sleepiness improved, but cataplexy continued. Her sleep physician later prescribed Xyrem which nearly abolished cataplexic episodes. In combination with good sleep hygiene practices, these medications produced a drastic decline in Felicia's daytime sleepiness. Her Epworth Sleepiness Scale score dropped from 19 to 10 after treatment and she was able to enjoy her time away from work once again.

Chapter 7

Restless Legs Syndrome

Life is something that happens when you can't get to sleep.
—**Fran Lebowitz**

Restless legs syndrome is characterized by a strong, often irresistible urge to move the legs. This is often accompanied by sensations such as tingling, numbness, or pain. Symptoms usually begin in the evening and are relieved by moving, stretching, or rubbing the legs.

Maria

Maria settles into her favorite reclining chair to unwind each night with every intention of completely relaxing. She reads a few more chapters in her book and channel-surfs until she lands on a sitcom that requires only as much brainpower as she has left after a long day. Eventually, Maria's tension melts and her body begins to relax.

But her legs are hardly at ease..

During the past few years, Maria has experienced uncomfortable sensations in her lower limbs. Her legs ache and tingle, and the sensations don't fade until she massages her legs, flexes her calves, or finally gets up and walks around her living room. Like clockwork, when her brain turns off for the day, her legs turn on. More worrisome is that recently she's noticed that the cramping surfaces for a minute or two during the day as well.

Once Maria retires to bed, the bothersome feeling prevents her from falling asleep and wakes her several times during the night.

The sensations stop only when she shimmies the lower half of her body, wiggles her toes, or gets out of bed and paces around the room. Her husband jokingly calls her "Twinkle Toes" because he feels her restless legs when he stretches out beside her in bed and hears her footsteps as she paces though the house during the night.

Maria's Sleep Assessment

Sleep snapshot

Once a sound sleeper, Maria developed insomnia two years ago with the onset of menopause. During the past six months, her condition has worsened. Her sleep is variable: she goes to bed anytime between 8:30 and 11 P.M. and usually spends an hour tossing and turning before she falls asleep. She wakes at least five times during the night. She assumes she is waking because she has to go to the bathroom, but she usually finds that her legs are uncomfortable and she must stretch or move them. Sometimes, she awakens because of hot flashes, although these have significantly lessened lately. Frustrated, Maria finally starts her day between 5 and 9 A.M. Her average five to six hours of sleep is far less than the eight to nine hours she could count on just five years ago. Because her nights are filled with frequent interruptions, she feels as if she never actually sleeps.

Excessive daytime sleepiness

Maria usually drags herself out of bed on weekday mornings to get ready for work. A nap is a luxury she can't afford to take, but sometimes she'll sneak in a short one—usually a quick 10 to 20 minutes during her lunch break.

Medical and family history

Maria does not report a family history of narcolepsy, sleep apnea, or other sleep disorders. However, she says her mother complained of feelings in her legs that kept her up at night.

Insomnia Maria has been taking prescription sleeping pills to treat her insomnia symptoms. She reports a significant amount of stress, and notes that her sleeplessness has worsened and that she is relying more on the medication. She takes it when she feels "really bad," which is at least once a week.

The diagnosis

Maria's physician asked her a series of questions about her sleep and ordered a polysomnogram to uncover the cause of her nighttime awakenings. He diagnosed her with restless legs syndrome (RLS). The time of day when Maria's legs bother her—in the early evening and during the night—is consistent with symptoms of RLS. Moreover, Maria's family history of RLS increased the likelihood by up to ten times that she might have the disorder.

All about Restless Legs Syndrome

Because symptoms of restless legs syndrome are often difficult to describe and may occur only once or twice per month at first, many people forget to bring up the subject when they see their doctor. Patients also routinely attribute the tingling in their legs to a pinched nerve from sitting in a particular body position or leg cramps. Others attribute the sensation to arthritis pain, vascular problems, or nervous system problems. Diabetics and people with kidney failure are particularly prone to RLS. Children who complain of achy legs are often brushed off by their parents' explanation that the sensations are growing pains. On top of this, patients might not recognize that tingling legs can trigger insomnia. But it's clear that when you aren't comfortable, you don't sleep.

Leg cramps or charley horses (sharp calf pains usually attributed to sore muscles or a mineral deficiency) are not the same as restless legs syndrome. If you have RLS, you may have a strong urge to move your legs at night—an urge you cannot resist. The feeling generally subsides in the morning, although patients with severe conditions report that sensations occasionally flare up during the day as well. The urge is often accompanied by a feeling of burning, itching, prickling, tingling, or aching, and the discomfort can range from mild to severe. Temporary relief comes only with moving the legs.

People afflicted with RLS sometimes also find that their leg muscles tighten or flex while they are still. Repetitive muscle movements in the lower extremities, known as periodic limb movements (PLMs), can occur during the night, arousing you and reducing quality of sleep. These movements also can occur while you are awake in bed. PLMs take center stage in another closely related disorder, known as periodic limb movement disorder (PLMD), which is characterized by periodic, repetitive limb movements during sleep that lead to insomnia or daytime sleepiness.

Periodic limb movement disorder and restless legs syndrome are two different sleep disorders. However, symptoms sometimes overlap, and about 85 percent of patients with RLS report involuntary leg jerking or twitching either during sleep or while they are still awake but sitting or lying in bed. Patients who are diagnosed with PLMD alone do not experience the type of sensations or level of discomfort associated with RLS.

Who gets RLS?

Restless legs syndrome has been described as the most common disorder no one has heard of. Between 5 and 10 percent of Caucasians in the world are affected. The disorder is rare among Asian populations. Restless legs syndrome is more common in women than in men, and it affects individuals of all ages. People who develop RLS before age 45 are considered early-onset cases and experience the onset of symptoms slowly over time. Once a person is 45 to 65 years old, RLS can set in suddenly and progress quickly. A patient might feel leg sensations every night from the day RLS starts.

More than 50 percent of patients with the disorder are diagnosed with primary or idiopathic RLS, meaning their restless legs are not associated with other medical problems. Many patients also report family histories of RLS or describe a parent who experienced unusual sensations and discomfort in the lower extremities. The chance of developing RLS increases ten-fold when an immediate relative has the disorder.

RLS and its relationship with other medical disorders A laundry list of medical problems and medications can produce the onset of RLS. There are links between the disorder and low levels of iron or anemia, Parkinson's disease, kidney failure, diabetes, and peripheral neuropathy (a nervous system disease). Pregnant women often note symptoms of RLS typically after 20 weeks of gestation, and dialysis patients are especially susceptible to developing RLS. If you take antidepressants, sedating antihistamines, antipsychotic medications, and virtually any centrally active dopamine-receptor antagonist (such as antinausea medication), you are a candidate for secondary RLS.

In many of these cases, RLS is a temporary disorder that is resolved when other conditions are treated. But when RLS regularly disturbs sleep, specific treatment methods are necessary.

How do I know I have RLS?

The hallmark of RLS is an intense, irresistible urge to move the legs, often accompanied by other sensations in the legs that may be difficult for you to describe. Certain criteria are necessary to make an RLS diagnosis. Patients must answer *yes* to the following questions:

1. Do you have the urge to move your extremities, usually accompanied by uncomfortable or unpleasant sensations in your legs?

2. Do you have the urge to move or have uncomfortable sensations that begin or worsen during periods of rest or inactivity?

3. Do you have the urge to move or have uncomfortable sensations that are partially or totally relieved by movement, such as walking or stretching?

4. Do you have the urge to move or have uncomfortable sensations that worsen or occur solely in the evening or at night?

There are some caveats to diagnosing patients with RLS using these criteria as the disorder changes naturally over time. These include:

- The patient previously met criteria for a diagnosis of RLS and has undergone a spontaneous remission or has received treatment producing significant alteration of symptoms.

- The patient at one time got relief of symptoms by activity, but discomfort now is so severe that relief is impossible.

- The patient at one time was worse later in the day or at night, but symptoms now are so severe that they are equal day and night.

If a patient presents with symptoms of RLS, a physician may use a standardized questionnaire, known as the International RLS Rating Scale, to grade the severity of the symptoms. Patients circle

The International RLS Rating Scale

If you think you may have RLS, please complete the following questionnaire based on how you have felt *during the past week*. Then, add up the numbers and use the scale given at the end of the test to see where you fall on the scale.

1. *Overall,* how would you rate the RLS *discomfort in your legs or arms?*

   (4) Very severe

   (3) Severe

   (2) Moderate

   (1) Mild

   (0) None

2. *Overall,* how would you rate the *need to move* around because of your RLS symptoms?

   (4) Very severe

   (3) Severe

   (2) Moderate

   (1) Mild

   (0) None

3. *Overall,* how much *relief of* your RLS arm or leg discomfort do you get from moving around?

   (4) No relief

   (3) Mild relief

   (2) Moderate relief

   (1) Either complete or almost complete relief

   (0) No RLS symptoms to be relieved

   (continued)

4. How severe was your *sleep disturbance* due to your RLS symptoms?

(4) Very severe

(3) Severe

(2) Moderate

(1) Mild

(0) None

5. How severe was your *tiredness* or *sleepiness* during the day due to your RLS symptoms?

(4) Very severe

(3) Severe

(2) Moderate

(1) Mild

(0) None

6. How severe was *your RLS as a whole*?

(4) Very severe

(3) Severe

(2) Moderate

(1) Mild

(0) None

7. How *often* did you get RLS symptoms?

(4) Very often (6–7 days a week)

(3) Often (4–5 days a week)

(2) Sometimes (2–3 days a week)

(1) Occasionally (1 day a week)

(0) Never

(continued)

8. When you had RLS symptoms, how severe were they on average?

(4) Very severe (8 hours or more per 24-hour day)

(3) Severe (3–8 hours per 24-hour day)

(2) Moderate (1–3 hours per 24-hour day)

(1) Mild (less than 1 hour per 24-hour day)

(0) None

9. *Overall*, how severe was the impact of your RLS symptoms on your ability to carry out your *daily affairs*—for example, carrying out a satisfactory family, home, social, school, or work life?

(4) Very severe

(3) Severe

(2) Moderate

(1) Mild

(0) None

10. How severe was your *mood disturbance* from your RLS symptoms—for example, angry, depressed, sad, anxious, or irritable?

(4) Very severe

(3) Severe

(2) Moderate

(1) Mild

(0) None

Severity Scale:

Very Severe	=	31–40 points
Severe	=	21–30 points
Moderate	=	11–20 points
Mild	=	1–10 points
None	=	0 points

the rating that describes how they felt during the past week. Physicians add the numbers to determine score of severity.

The Polysomnogram

A diagnosis of RLS is made using a patient's sleep history. In this case, overnight sleep testing is not necessarily required. Maria, however, was referred to a sleep lab to evaluate the repeated awakenings she experienced nearly every night. Maria's overnight sleep study demonstrated a delayed sleep onset during which she squirmed and exercised her legs in bed, trying to relieve the sensation. Periods of leg stretching were punctuated by involuntary leg jerks. Once asleep, her legs continued to jerk repeatedly during intervals of light sleep and during the transition from wakefulness to sleep. Movements lessened during deep NREM sleep and were absent in REM sleep.

How to Get a Good Night's Sleep

A regular exercise program can reduce symptoms of RLS in patients with mild cases. Movement during the day has been shown to ease leg sensations in the evening. While sitting, patients with less advanced RLS can reduce symptoms by staying mentally active.

General measures

Symptoms of RLS can be lessened by taking these steps:

- Reduce caffeine intake
- Limit use of alcohol
- Stop smoking
- Eliminate drugs known to cause RLS

When symptoms of RLS occur, the following activities can alleviate sensations:

- Walking
- Riding an exercise bike
- Massaging or rubbing lower leg area
- Soaking in a hot tub

Because iron deficiency is a reversible cause of RLS, many sleep specialists recommend over-the-counter iron tablets (ferrous sulfate). A simple blood test can measure iron stores in the body and determine who might benefit from iron therapy. Iron is typically administered one to three times a day along with vitamin C, which increases its absorption. Treatment should continue for several months or until iron levels normalize. Constipation is common side effect of iron therapy and may require treatment by increasing dietary fiber content or the use of a stool softener.

Medications

Physicians can treat RLS with four different classes of medications depending on the severity of RLS, possible side effects and interactions with other medications a patient may be taking, and whether symptoms are painful. In recent years, dopaminergic drugs that replace dopamine, a neurotransmitter in the brain have been increasingly used to treat RLS. Also used for conditions such as Parkinson's disease, these drugs control the urge to move and sensory symptoms and reduce involuntary leg jerking during sleep. Currently, ropinirole (Requip) and pramipraxole (Mirapex) are the only FDA-approved drugs for RLS.

Four classes of drugs are available to treat RLS:

Dopaminergic drugs: These are the primary therapies used to treat moderate to severe RLS in patients who are unresponsive to non-drug interventions. Included in this class of drugs are ropinirole, pramipexole, and levodopa. Levodopa is best suited to treat people with intermittent RLS because continuous use is associated with augmentation. A phenomenon seen less commonly with ropinirole and pramiprexole, *augmentation* is most common with levodopa. Patients with augmentation experience symptoms with increased intensity earlier in the day, such as in the early evening, in the afternoon hours, or even in the morning. In other cases, symptoms become more intense over the course of the day, or affect other parts of the body. Maintaining the lowest effective dose of dopaminergic drugs reduces the development of augmentation. The most common side effects of these agents include nausea, headache, hallucinations, and hypotension.

Antiseizure medications: These drugs control sensations by slowing or blocking pain signals from nerves. Examples include gabapentin, carbamazepine, and pregabalin. Gabapentin and pregabalin are particularly effective in patients with painful RLS related to peripheral nervous system disorders. These agents are generally well-tolerated. Side effects include sleepiness, dizziness, and weight gain.

Benzodiazepines: Sometimes prescribed for RLS, these drugs are generally not considered first-line treatments because of their addictive potential and side effects like daytime drowsiness. Clonazepam and temazepam fall into this category.

Opioids: These painkiller drugs are used to alleviate aching and uncomfortable sensations in the legs of patients with RLS. Because of their potential for addiction, they are usually reserved for treating more severe cases that are not controlled with other agents and cases of painful RLS. Opioids are controlled substances that usually require a special type of prescription. Many opioids are available, including codeine, oxycodone, propoxyphene, morphine, and methadone, which is reserved for the most severe cases.

Maria's Outcome

The physician ordered a blood test to rule out iron deficiency, and Maria's results were normal. He then recommended a trial of ropinirole, beginning with one pill at 8 P.M. The dose was timed to coincide with the onset of Maria's leg movements, which usually started by 10 P.M. (One problem that often leads to incomplete response to treatment is that medications are often taken too late in the evening. If you have symptoms in the early evening, you should take your first dose of medication at dinnertime.)

Maria's doctor increased the dose gradually, until the medication abolished virtually all symptoms and Maria's quality of sleep improved. He warned her about the possibility of developing augmentation, a phenomenon in which symptoms of RLS begin earlier in the day because of the treatment. He also warned her about unusual side effects, including sudden sleep attacks and melanoma, a rare complication of dopaminergic therapy observed in patients with Parkinson's disease.

In Maria's case, treating her RLS allowed her to sleep seven and sometimes even eight hours each night, reducing her daytime sleepiness and decreasing the number of night awakenings. Once in a while, particularly after a long, stressful day, Maria still notices that same familiar achy feeling and finds herself repositioning herself in bed to find a comfortable spot. Thankfully, though, she remains free of RLS symptoms during the day.

Chapter 8

Psychophysiological Insomnia

Insomnia is a gross feeder. It will nourish itself on any kind of thinking, including thinking about not thinking.
—Clifton Fadiman

Psychophysiological insomnia occurs when a patient responds to stress or other environmental conditions with tension. The patient learns sleep-preventing associations, which result in difficulty falling and staying asleep.

Ann

Ann recalls her worst string of sleepless nights—40 in a row. She dreads turning the light out at night because she knows that she probably won't nod off until at least 2 A.M. Faced with the prospect of yet another sleepless night, she turns to worrying and her nightly pep talk before going to bed. Tonight, you can sleep, she tells herself. But what if I can't sleep? How long will I stay awake tonight? How can I lose sleep another night? It's already getting late . . . .

Once in bed, Ann lies awake, subtracting each passing hour from the sleep total she should achieve before her 6 A.M. wake-up call for work. It's a numbers game for Ann, and the more minutes she counts, the more sleep she loses. While she's awake, she can't stop thinking about her sick in-laws, her work responsibilities, and her changing body, which won't let her feel "normal." How will I hold it all together? she frets.

Just before the onset of this particular bout of insomnia, Ann's doctor had changed her sleeping-pill prescription. The new medication didn't seem to be working, so Ann attributed her current insomnia to not being able to adjust to the different prescription. Ann had been anxious about the switch. But she was uneasy about a lot of things in her life these days.

Ann, 46, has complained of insomnia for the past six years. Symptoms of perimenopause and related physical changes, including hot flashes or night sweats, disrupt her sleep from time to time. But lately, the wakefulness has lasted between two and three hours on "really bad" nights. During a sleep assessment, Ann mentioned that a few years ago she was treated for depression. When the physician pressed her for details, Ann said she had worked through that period of her life.

Ann has taken some steps to improve her sleep environment. She removed the television from her bedroom—a distraction that can trigger insomnia. She also established a nighttime ritual. But her disruptive sleep is also a regular pattern, and Ann estimates that she sleeps only four hours each night.

Ann's Sleep Assessment

Sleep snapshot

Ann spends eight hours in bed each night, but she thinks only four hours are spent sleeping. She estimates that she needs eight hours to function properly. She goes to bed at 10 P.M. and wakes at 6 A.M. each morning. She maintains a relatively consistent sleep schedule on weekends, indulging in several extra hours in bed on Saturdays and Sundays, but during this time she rarely does more than rest. Ann avoids eating, watching television, or reading in bed. She knows that poor sleep hygiene will only worsen her ability to sleep at night. She consistently wakes several times per night, sometimes every hour on the hour. Just before and during her menstrual period, she usually spends at least one night entirely sleepless, or so it seems.

Ann takes a prescription sleeping pill as needed at bedtime. In fact, she has seen several physicians for her sleep problem and has taken just about every prescription sleeping pill on the market. Most didn't work for more than a few days, but Ann is afraid to go without her nightly pill. It has become a security blanket. She also takes a number of vitamins, including calcium, vitamins C, B, and E, and a soy supplement.

Excessive daytime sleepiness

Ann never feels refreshed. She is always tired and fatigued, and she couldn't nap during the day if her life depended on it. She is growing more concerned that her sleep loss will become apparent to her boss or that she'll fall asleep while she is driving. She also worries that her sleepless nights are jeopardizing her health. She wonders how long a human being can survive without sleep.

Medical and family history

Ann is healthy, although she exhibited some atypical chest pain a couple of years ago. This pain was a normal reaction to stress. She says her family does not have a history of narcolepsy, restless legs syndrome, or insomnia. She told the physician that her father died when she was 13 years old. After this, she had fears of being separated from her mother that led to some sleepless nights which passed with time.

Restless legs syndrome Once a month, Ann develops an ache in her calf that increases when she puts weight on her leg. This can happen day or night, and she usually controls the discomfort by applying a heating pad to the area or doing squats to stretch her lower leg muscles. Nevertheless, the sensation is uncomfortable and can inhibit sleep. Ann has never been treated for an iron deficiency, which is associated with uncomfortable legs and restless legs syndrome.

Narcolepsy Ann does not nap during the day, and though she often is worn out from restless nights, she is alert and scored a 4 on the Epworth Sleepiness Scale. (Remember, Felicia's score was 19; she had narcolepsy. Scores of 10 and higher indicate daytime sleepiness.)

Insomnia When the physician asked Ann about recent changes or life events, he learned about her father's untimely death many years earlier and stresses related to her job and marriage that keep her awake at night. Ann denies being depressed, though she said hormonal changes have made her anxious lately. The emotional activity in Ann's life spurred the doctor to explore potential psychophysiological insomnia, which develops because of two factors: somatized tension (muscle movement) and perpetuating behaviors that are disruptive to sleep (ruminating, worrying, and so forth). Her Fatigue Severity Score is 56 out of a maximum of 63, indicating a pronounced degree of fatigue and lack of energy.

Bruxism Ann's husband noticed that she sometimes grinds her teeth during the night. Ann has a mouth guard, but she often does not wear it. If her jaw hurts in the morning, she will rub the area, take some ibuprofen, or use a heating pad. Her teeth grinding worsens during stressful times. This type of nervous activity is not unusual for insomniacs.

The diagnosis

Ann is shouldering a great deal of stress in her life, her body is going through midlife change, and her emotions are responding to these internal and external factors through anxiety. Pulled in several directions, Ann is like many women who try to "hold it all together." Women are more likely to have insomnia than men, and women in Ann's age group are even more susceptible to the sleep disorder, because their hormones are affecting their ability to get a good night's sleep. (The *Cleveland Clinic Guide to Menopause*, by Dr. Holly L. Thacker, addresses the effects of hormonal changes on sleep in more detail and offers solutions for midlife women who have trouble sleeping.)

When the physician learned about Ann's history of depression, he questioned whether this was still an issue. Ann said that problems

Are you sleepy or fatigued?

While not everyone perceives a difference, distinguishing sleepiness from fatigue is useful in the diagnosis of sleep disorders. Signs and symptoms of excessive sleepiness are:

- Yawning during the day
- Struggling to keep your eyes open during sedentary situations
- Head nodding
- Ability to nap when given the opportunity

In contrast, fatigued patients often report:

- Lack of energy
- Inability to exercise or accomplish tasks due to tiredness
- Difficulty falling asleep despite feelings of sheer physical and mental exhaustion
- Feeling as exhausted after waking up in the morning as they did the night before

in her marriage five years ago prompted her to see a psychologist to discuss ways to cope with tension. She took a prescription antidepressant for a short time. Because Ann had difficulty coping with stress in the past, the physician linked this past behavior with her response to the family challenges she faced today.

Ann isn't losing sleep because of idiopathic insomnia, which is a lifelong insomnia not caused by stress or emotional disturbances. She has experienced difficulty falling asleep only in recent years, so the physician knows that her disorder did not develop during childhood as a result of an inadequately developed sleep system or neurological disorder. Rather, Ann's insomnia flared because of psychological and physical reasons. The physician's clinical impression of Ann was that she suffered from psychophysiological insomnia. The root of Ann's sleeping problems is not intrinsic, but rather a reaction to outside influences. Ann's restless sleep is learned, the physician told her. It can be treated by cognitive behavioral therapy and improved sleep hygiene.

Why Can't I Sleep?

There are universal triggers that keep people awake at night.

Medical conditions, even temporary ones such as a sprained ankle, a sports injury, or minor surgery, can prevent sound sleep. Chronic problems, such as heartburn, asthma, heart disease, pain disorders, and arthritis, can also cause insomnia.

Life changes (a baby, a new spouse, a new job) figure into the sleep equation. Many of these changes are exciting or present new challenges. Until you settle comfortably into new relationships and roles, sleep can suffer.

Emotions can inhibit sleep. When we feel frustration or anger, anticipation, or even happiness, we tend to stay awake long past bedtime. Divorce, loss of a loved one, major illness, lawsuits, and bad investments produce negative emotions and promote anxiety—not states of mind that lead to relaxation and restful nights.

About Insomnia

Insomnia is among the most common complaints adults report to their doctors and an important, often unrecognized, public health issue. It can significantly impair a person's ability to function safely and effectively in social and occupational situations and can hinder quality of life. The economic costs of insomnia in the U.S.—a tally that includes increased health care utilization, decreased productivity, absenteeism, and occupational and motor vehicle accidents—is staggering. A 1995 study estimated the total cost of insomnia, including appointments with doctors and psychologists and hospital care, to be just under $14 billion.

The word *insomnia* describes difficulty initiating sleep, maintaining sleep, early awakening, or nonrestorative sleep despite adequate opportunity for sleep. The disorder is accompanied by at least one of the following forms of daytime impairment:

- Fatigue or daytime sleepiness
- Attention, concentration, or memory impairment
- Poor social, occupational, or academic performance
- Mood disturbance or irritability
- Reduction in motivation, energy, or initiative
- Proneness for errors and/or accidents at work or while driving
- Tension headaches or gastrointestinal distress
- Worries about sleep

Who gets insomnia?

Insomnia is the most common sleep complaint. In the 2005 National Sleep Foundation's Sleep in America Poll, approximately half the population surveyed reported insomnia. Respondents reported at least one symptom of insomnia for at least a few nights per week during the prior year. Insomnia is more common in women and adults over 65 years of age. People with mental health disorders including depression and anxiety are particularly vulnerable as are patients with chronic medical problems (see below).

How do I know if I have insomnia?

To determine if you have insomnia, ask yourself the following questions:

- Does it take you an excessively long period of time to fall asleep?

- Do you wake frequently? If so, do you have a difficult time falling asleep again?

- Do you notice that although you have difficulty falling asleep at night, you fall asleep easily during sedentary activities, such as watching television or reading?

- Do you watch television, read, or eat in bed?

- Are you a worrywart? Does your mind race at night? Do you spend the nighttime hours thinking about your problems, the next day's schedule, or worries about sleep loss?

- Do you experience increased muscle tension or agitation (conditions known to sleep professionals as somatized tension) or inability to relax at night?

- Have you experienced a recent life change or emotional stress?

- Do you feel anxious or depressed?

- Do you complain of not sleeping? Do you grow tired or irritable, or feel a deterioration of mood or motivation, during the day?

If you answered *yes* to any of these questions, consider visiting a physician to discuss sleep patterns and solutions. The physician will ask you to maintain a sleep log in which you track bedtimes, hours asleep, and how you feel during the day. The information you collect is important to determine how your sleep compares with "normal" sleep.

If your sleep has been disrupted for more than a month and interferes with how you function during the day, you should talk to your physician or ask for a referral to see a sleep disorders specialist.

What causes insomnia?

Most people experience brief periods in their lives when they can't sleep—this is normal. But when sleepless behavior persists for a month or longer, and lack of sleep interferes with a person's ability to function during the day, the problem is more serious and warrants changes in lifestyle or cognitive behavioral therapy. To determine the best course of action, physicians must understand the cause of the insomnia. Several reasons—intrinsic and extrinsic—can cause people to lose sleep.

Diet Caffeinated substances, including coffee, tea, soda, and chocolate, over-the-counter wakefulness-promoting agents, and some prescription drugs, stimulate the nervous system and may cause difficulty falling asleep or cause you to wake up during the night. This is not to say you should take your morning coffee off the breakfast menu or forget your late-afternoon chocolate. Consuming moderate amounts of caffeine during the day will not affect sleep onset in the evening for most people, particularly if they curb consumption several hours before bedtime. If you suffer from insomnia, limit your intake of caffeinated beverages after noon. Excessive caffeine use can lead to withdrawal symptoms, which can also affect a person's ability to sleep.

Nicotine is another sleep-inhibiting stimulant. Smokers who break their habit might experience withdrawal symptoms at first, but once their body adjusts, they will find that they wake up less often and sleep more soundly at night. If you can't quit the habit entirely, avoid smoking in the evening and absolutely during the night.

Despite the theory that a nightcap is just the elixir to bring about a good night's sleep, alcoholic beverages actually interfere with the body's ability to maintain deep sleep, which refreshes the body. Alcohol might induce sleep at first, but regular consumers are likely to wake up frequently and often report feeling drowsy and sleep-deprived in the morning.

Finally, full meals before bedtime can trigger heartburn and stomachache—two reasons to eat heavy meals no later than four hours before going to sleep. A light snack, on the other hand, can promote sleep. Milk or cheese and crackers are good bedtime snacks.

Environment: your bedroom Some insomniacs set themselves up for a sleepless night before they even attempt to close their eyes. Rather than a calming oasis that promotes sleep and relaxation, their bedrooms are activity centers equipped with televisions, computers, stereos, books, magazines, and other distractions. Still other sleep-inhibiting stimulation may be attributed to noise that's no fault of their own. Perhaps their windows don't close out noise from a crowded street, their home is located under a flight path, a train passes every morning at 3 A.M., or they can hear their neighbor's stereo thumping all night in the apartment next door.

Of course, it is unrealistic to assume that every bedroom can be converted into a cocoon that blocks out all light, sound, and activity. You can't stop the train, and you probably won't move just because of the airport. (Noisy neighbors, on the other hand, might be reason to break a lease). A number of distractions are beyond your control, but for the sake of a good night's sleep, you can eliminate quite a few sleep-inhibiting factors.

You might not realize that environmental stresses are keeping you awake. Consider the hard-working executive who thinks checking e-mail on his laptop while propped up on his pillow in bed is a way to get ahead of tomorrow's work. Bringing work to bed introduces into the bedroom the same behaviors, feelings, and stresses he might feel when he's in the office. Turn off your e-mail well before bedtime, and don't grade papers, read reports, review presentations, or double-check the financials while you are curled up under the sheets. Save your work for the morning, or at least corral it in an office or another room. Separate work and sleep. If you find yourself mentally active and worrying in bed, set aside some time in the late afternoon or early evening to review tomorrow's to-do list so you can get it out of the way before you retire.

The number of environmental stimulants is large and not limited to work or work-related stresses. Some insomniacs, for example, watch television as they doze off, claiming that the white noise calms them. This might be true. But the sounds are also jarring and can disrupt sleep-stage transitions and overall sleep. Eating in bed is yet another bad habit that insomniacs should break. Even a bedroom clock can keep you from sleeping, as in Ann's obsession with counting the minutes until her alarm sounded. This is a common problem for insomniacs. If you notice that you worry about the time, try sleeping with your alarm clock facing the other direction. Sleeping without time pressure is easier than playing the time game.

Insomnia and sleep insecurity In addition to anxiety, depression, or underlying psychological disorders already present in many patients diagnosed with various types of insomnia, patients like Ann develop a fear of not falling asleep. You may worry each night. *What if I can't fall asleep? How will I function at my meeting tomorrow on two hours of rest? Will tonight be as bad as last night?* Then you might feverishly check the glaring, digitized numbers on your clock or turn on the television to distract yourself. Sleep insecurity grows with every toss and turn, with every night of lost sleep.

Like most patients who exhibit symptoms of insomnia, Ann subscribes to a nightly pattern. Her insomnia was triggered by a combination of stress and physical change that included the onset

Medical and Psychiatric Disorders Associated with Insomnia

A variety of medical and psychiatric conditions and their treatment can cause insomnia. Insomnia caused by psychosocial stressors, medications, psychiatric and medical disorders, and drug or substance abuse is referred to as *secondary insomnia.*

The disorders and conditions that can trigger a diagnosis of secondary insomnia include:

Psychiatric disorders
Mood disorders: Depression, bipolar disorder, dysthymia
Anxiety disorders: Generalized anxiety disorder, panic disorder, post-traumatic stress disorder
Psychotic disorders: Paranoia, schizophrenia, delusional disorder

Medical disorders
Cardiovascular: Angina, heart failure
Respiratory: Chronic obstructive pulmonary disease, asthma
Neurologic: Alzheimer's disease, Parkinson's disease
Rheumatic: Fibromyalgia, chronic fatigue syndrome, osteoarthritis
Gastrointestinal: Gastroesophageal reflux disease, irritable bowel syndrome
Sleep: Restless legs syndrome, sleep apnea, circadian rhythm disorders

Drug and substance abuse
Alcohol
Tobacco
Recreational drugs
Caffeine

Prescription medications
Beta blockers
Steroids
Levodopa
Stimulants
Thyroid hormone

of: menopause, difficulties in her marriage, and ill family members. Some people react to tension by getting headaches, stomachaches, or other physical maladies, but people like Ann respond by not sleeping.

People feed their own disorder by developing habits that disrupt sleep. Essentially, the insecurity that diagnosed insomniacs feel when they try to sleep worsens the disorder and increases their sleep deficit. They are not relaxed in the evening, so they watch television or read in bed to fall asleep, but the television or book distracts them, so they remain wide awake during the night. Because they are tired during the day, they turn to caffeine and other stimulants, which can trigger wakefulness hours after the substances are consumed. It becomes a vicious cycle.

Are there different kinds of insomnia?

The different types of insomnia are classified based on the age of the patient at symptom onset (some cases start early in life) and duration of symptoms, and each type may be attributable to different causes and triggers. It is important for your doctor to determine which type of insomnia you may be suffering from in order to properly treat you.

Acute insomnia Also referred to as adjustment insomnia, this short-term insomnia is the most common sleep problem. It occurs when a situational stress temporarily disrupts sleep. Transient insomnia can progress into permanent insomnia if sleeplessness persists for more than a few months and the person cannot break the cycle. Some triggers for adjustment insomnia include final exams, a surgical procedure, or a new job.

Chronic insomnia In long-term insomnias, difficulty falling asleep or staying asleep occurs more than a few nights per week for a period of at least six months. More than 70 million Americans complain of insomnia, according to the National Institutes of Health, and many different reasons can be responsible for keeping diagnosed individuals awake all night. Visiting a physician or sleep disorders specialist is especially important to treating chronic insomnia. Through the sleep and medical history, sleep questionnaires, and a polysomnogram in select cases, insomniacs can determine whether there are underlying causes for their problem (such as sleep apnea or restless legs syndrome).

Psychophysiological insomnia Psychophysiological insomnia can start innocently, perhaps with a lack of sleep for a few nights. Then the problem escalates into a pattern. Lost sleep intrudes on your lifestyle, affecting mood, motivation, performance, and energy level.

Ann is a classic case of psychophysiological insomnia. Some of the typical features of this form of insomnia are:

- Excessive focus on sleep or heightened anxiety levels about sleep

- Difficulty falling asleep in bed at the desired time, but not during sedentary activities that take place at other times of day

- Ability to fall asleep better away from home

- Mental arousal in bed (racing thoughts, inability to turn off an active mind)

- Heightened physical tension in bed (inability to relax)

Ann reacted to stress by not sleeping. Her pattern evolved into a lifestyle of losing sleep, and the fatigue further affected her mood and outlook. Soon, bedtime was a greater stress than the emotional tension in her life, and sleeping became an impossible feat—something she feared each night.

Individuals with psychophysiological insomnia might deny the impact that stressful events have on them or their feelings of depression and anxiety. They blame insomnia for their lack of sleep, rather than correctly placing responsibility for their sleeplessness on the events currently taking place in their lives. Insomnia becomes learned, and a vicious cycle develops. The hallmark of psychophysiological insomnia is a person's focus and near obsession with the sleep problem. This attention contributes to sleep loss.

Fifteen percent of people seen in sleep centers are diagnosed with psychophysiological insomnia, which affects 1 to 2 percent of adults. Onset of psychophysiological insomnia generally occurs in midlife or surrounding a major life stressor (job loss, medical problem, death in family, divorce), and the problem occurs more frequently in women. It gradually escalates until patients seek treatment.

Note: A diagnosis of psychophysiological insomnia is not made in patients who are diagnosed with anxiety syndromes, phobias, obsessive-compulsive neurosis, major depression, or other psychopathologies. Sleep problems associated with these psychiatric disorders should be treated as part of the psychiatric disorder.

The Polysomnogram

Because insomnia is usually diagnosed based on sleep history, most patients do not require a polysomnogram. However, laboratory testing should be considered for both patients who are experiencing insomnia in addition to symptoms of sleep apnea or periodic limb movement disorder, and patients with typical symptoms who fail to improve with standard treatment. A polysomnogram of a patient diagnosed with psychophysiological insomnia may show prolonged time taken to fall asleep (sleep latency), an increase in stage 1 sleep, and a decrease in stage 3 sleep (delta or deep sleep), along with frequent arousals. However, sometimes these patients sleep better in the laboratory or a hotel or friend's house than at home.

How to Get a Good Night's Sleep

Insomnia is more than just a nighttime nuisance. Chronic insomnia can cause significant emotional distress, fatigue, sleepiness, and impairment of daytime functioning. Interpersonal relationships and work performance may be affected and a person's quality of life can quickly deteriorate. Individuals with insomnia have a higher rate of mental health problems, drug and alcohol abuse, heart problems, painful muscle and joint conditions, and health care utilization (more trips to the doctor and greater chance of ending up in the hospital). There is strong evidence linking insomnia and depression and, to a lesser extent, insomnia with anxiety disorders. Insomnia increases a person's risk of occupational injuries, motor vehicle accidents, and even death.

Following are some tips for getting a good night's sleep:

Practicing good sleep hygiene

- Sleep only when you are drowsy.

- If you cannot fall or stay asleep, leave your bedroom and read or engage in a relaxing activity in another room.

- Do not allow yourself to fall asleep outside the bedroom; return to the bed to rest.

- Maintain regular wake times.

- Use your bedroom only for sleep and intimate relations.

- Avoid napping during the day. (If you're extremely exhausted, limit naps to less than one hour, no later than 3 p.m.)

- Avoid caffeine within four to six hours of bedtime.

- Avoid nicotine close to bedtime and during the night.

- Do not drink alcoholic beverages within four to six hours of bedtime.

- Avoid large meals; limit yourself to a small snack before bedtime.

- Avoid strenuous exercise within a few hours of going to sleep.

- Minimize light, noise, and extreme temperatures in the bedroom.

Behavioral therapy

Improving sleep hygiene is the first step toward establishing a regimen that will promote sound sleep. But patients like Ann also benefit from cognitive behavior therapy. Cognitive behavior therapy, or CBT, is a broad term applied to a variety of techniques that are used to treat insomnia and other disorders. The goal of CBT is to empower patients and help them gain control over sleep through education. Cognitive behavior therapy corrects a patient's thought patterns and behaviors that can cause or worsen insomnia, and the approach is not only effective, but its benefits outlast over-the-counter and prescription treatments.

Cognitive behavior therapy is structured and focused treatment, and patients must play an active role to realize its benefits. A typical session lasts between 40 and 60 minutes and is usually conducted by a psychologist. The course of treatment varies from six to ten sessions, depending on the intensity of the problem and the patient's progress. There are two drawbacks to CBT: there are not enough professionals trained in CBT, and insurance coverage limits access for many patients. Given those restrictions, some insomniacs find ways to utilize the techniques on their own. It is also important to know from the start that no treatment will provide instant relief—particularly in cases of chronic insomnia. The trick is to work at it one step at a time, with the goal of eventually developing healthy sleep patterns.

Some of the benefits of CBT include:

- Increase in total sleep time
- Improved sleep efficiency
- Decrease in sleep latency (time it takes to fall asleep)
- Decrease in awakenings during the night

Following are various CBT practices that are used to correct problematic sleep patterns and reestablish positive thinking about sleep:

1. **Sleep restriction:** Most insomniacs stay in bed too long, frustrated and unable to fall asleep. Sleep restriction allows patients to spend only as much time in bed as they report sleeping (but no less than four hours). When sleep efficiency improves to 85 percent, time in bed is increased in 15- to 20-minute increments per night each week. If sleep efficiency falls below roughly 85 percent, the time spent in bed is decreased by the same amount.

2. **Relaxation training:** Meditation, progressive muscle relaxation (PMR), deep-breathing exercises, and guided imagery that calm the mind and body can help a patient slow down and prepare for sleep. Progressive muscle relaxation trains the patient to recognize and control tension by performing exercises that consist of first tensing and then relaxing a series of muscle groups. In deep-breathing exercises, patients are trained to inhale and exhale slowly as the abdomen expands and contracts. The goal is to learn how to breathe slowly and relax during anxiety-provoking situations. Guided imagery and meditation are used to focus the patient on pleasant thoughts instead of racing ones.

3. **Stimulus control:** Retraining a patient to see the bedroom as a relaxing place means using the room only for sleep and

intimate relations. If a patient is not sleeping, he or she must get out of bed and move to another room. A nightly bout of frustration only serves to associate the space with stress, thereby worsening insomnia. The idea is to make this room as peaceful as possible to promote sound sleep. Start by not letting yourself lay in bed for more than 20 minutes if you cannot sleep. Avoid thoughts and behaviors, such as watching the clock, that lead to mental activation or frustration while trying to fall asleep.

4. **Biofeedback:** Relaxation is the key. Biofeedback trains a patient to improve health by developing a greater awareness of and control over feelings of stress and anxiety. Depending on the technique, the level of stress and anxiety may be measured by placing electrodes or sensors on the scalp, the forehead, around the chest and abdomen, or on the fingertip to record biological signals. In neurofeedback, brain wave activity recorded from the scalp is visualized on the computer screen. The therapist assists the subject in relaxing, thereby increasing slower EEG frequencies that facilitate sleep. In respiratory biofeedback, sensors measure respiratory rate, rhythm, and volume. The patient sees and hears breathing patterns during anxiety. A therapist shows the patient how to modify breathing during stressful times. Similar techniques are used in thermal biofeedback (measuring changes in blood flow), muscle tension biofeedback, and other procedures.

Medication

Sleeping pills Ann's physician advised her to continue taking her sleeping-pill prescription, but to try to reduce usage over a period of six months first by reducing the dose and next by the number of nights of use. Sleeping pills are widely available today, and some newer formulations are less addictive and shorter acting than older drugs like valium, so the patients who take them don't feel hung over or drowsy the next day.

Sleeping pills can be used to break a bout of insomnia, get on track to improve sleep patterns, and achieve sounder sleep for a period of time, but these medications should be used as a temporary solution. Doctors can prescribe short- or long-acting drugs, depending on when a patient loses sleep. If falling asleep is the problem, short-acting drugs will facilitate sleep and prevent drowsy mornings. If maintaining sleep in the middle of the night is a concern, long-acting drugs provide relief. You should consult a doctor before using these or any type of sleep aid.

In addition to prescription sleeping pills, drugstores offer an array of over-the-counter sleep aids, though many insomniacs find these ineffective. Most of them consist of sedating antihistamines.

Many insomniacs rely on sleeping pills as a crutch; they can't sleep without them because they have a fixed idea that they need the drugs to be able to sleep. Without them, they worry that they will stay awake all night. (Remember Ann's anxiety when her doctor changed her sleeping-pill prescription? She worried that it would not work as well as her old standby.)

In most cases, sleeping pills are not a permanent solution, but they can help in the short term, particularly for patients with acute insomnia related to a sudden, unexpected life stressor and in situations that involve resetting a patient's body clock, including jet lag and shift-work schedule changes.

Benzodiazepine hypnotics Prior to the early 1990s, these were the drugs of choice to treat insomnia. More recently, however, research has shown that patients using benzodiazepine develop tolerance to the drug, dependence, and withdrawal. Benzodiazepines have a potential for significant side effects, including residual daytime sedation, cognitive impairment, motor incoordination, dizziness, low blood pressure, and respiratory depression (low respiratory rate). These agents should be used cautiously in people with a history of substance abuse, in the elderly, and in those with respiratory problems, such as chronic obstructive pulmonary disease and sleep apnea. Benzodiazepines are contraindicated in treating people with severe respiratory disorders. In the elderly, benzodiazepines are associated with an increased risk of hip fractures secondary to low blood pressure and falls. Use of these drugs to treat insomnia has declined with the introduction of safer alternatives.

Non-benzodiazepine hypnotics First introduced to the U.S. market in 1992, non-benzodiazepine hypnotics are an alternative to traditional benzodiazepines and are just as effective. Patients who take non-benzodiazepine hypnotics for insomnia notice decreased incidence of amnesia, daytime sleepiness, respiratory depression, orthostatic hypotension (feeling dizzy when standing or walking), and falls. However, these drugs are not entirely benign. In recent years, these drugs have been noted to cause sleepwalking, sleep-eating, and even sleep-driving in some patients.

Melatonin receptor agonists The first and only melatonin receptor agonist was approved by the FDA for the treatment of insomnia in July 2005. This drug acts selectively in the part of the brain that regulates the body's internal clock, thereby promoting sleep onset and maintenance of a circadian rhythm.

Ann's Outcome

Ann was evaluated by a sleep specialist and a psychologist with expertise in treating insomnia. She was asked to keep a sleep log to determine the regularity of her sleep-wake cycle. The specialist also instructed her to eliminate caffeine and set aside time each day to plan the next day.

The sleep logs proved very useful, and documented the many hours Ann was spending in bed awake, tossing and turning, which sparked frustration and fed her negative attitude about getting sleep. Her psychologist told her about the 20-minute toss-and-turn rule and instructed her to get out of bed if she'd been lying awake for 20 minutes or longer. Ann also learned how to use progressive muscle relaxation to clear her mind and distract her from negative sleep thoughts.

Ann's sleeping pill was continued initially. She returned to the psychologist for monthly visits to monitor progress and learned new behavioral strategies. Eventually, she was able to do without her sleeping pill (although she keeps it in the medicine cabinet for those nights that she just can't get to sleep on her own).

People with psychophysiological insomnia usually improve with treatment but rarely sleep as well as they recall sleeping in years past. Ann's motivation and persistence with treatment paid off. But in times of stress, or if she neglected to use the techniques she learned during cognitive behavioral therapy, her sleep quality would quickly revert to sleepless nights.

Following are some basic principles that should govern the use of sleeping pills.

- Tell your doctor about all your medical conditions and any other medications you are taking before he or she prescribes a sleeping pill.

- Sleeping pills are not used as the sole treatment for insomnia. Sleep hygiene and behavioral therapies should be also implemented.

- Sleeping pills are started at low doses and titrated slowly as needed.

- Never mix sleeping pills with alcohol or other central nervous system depressant medications.

- Take a sleeping pill only when you will have enough time (7 to 8 hours) to get a full night of sleep.

- Never drive a car or operate machinery after taking a sleeping pill.

- Long-term use of certain sleeping pills (like the benzodiazepines) should be avoided.

- Sleeping pills should be used cautiously by people with a history of substance abuse or dependence.

- Patients should be monitored regularly for tolerance, dependence, and withdrawal.

- Use of sleeping pills use should be tapered gradually to avoid withdrawal symptoms and rebound insomnia.

The following sleep aids are used to treat insomnia:

Prescription medications

Zolpidem (Ambien): Used for the short-term treatment of insomnia, this sleep aid decreases sleep latency and increases duration of sleep. Because of its rapid onset and short duration of action, it is best for sleep-onset insomnia, although a controlled-release form is also available.

Zaleplon (Sonata): This drugs's ultra-short half-life of one hour means it has no hangover effect. Used for short-term treatment of insomnia, it increases total sleep time and decreases awakenings. Best for sleep-onset insomnia; those with middle-of-the-night insomnia can take an extra dose because of its short duration of action.

Eszopiclone (Lunesta): Approved for long-term use, this sleep aid decreases sleep latency and wake time after sleep onset and increases sleep efficiency. It has a longer half-life (five to six hours), so it should be used when patients expect to spend at least eight hours in bed. It is effective for sleep-onset insomnia and sleep maintenance.

Ramelteon (Rozeram): Approved in 2005 for sleep-onset insomnia, ramelteon is the most recent addition to the market. It is the first prescription insomnia medication that binds to the brain's melatonin receptors, thereby facilitating sleep and maintaining normal circadian rhythms. It is the only prescription sleep aid that does not act by depressing the central nervous system. It is also the first insomnia drug that does not have abuse potential. Due to its short half-life, this drug is most effective for sleep-onset insomnia.

Antidepressants

Low doses of sedating antidepressants such as trazodone (Desyrel), amitriptyline (Elavil) and mirtazapine (Remeron), are often prescribed to non-depressed patients for the treatment of insomnia. But there is essentially no evidence to support this practice. These agents should be used sparingly for insomnia because of their limited efficacy and the potential for significant side effects.

Note: Dosage adjustments are usually required in seniors and people with liver impairment. All drugs require a prescription from a physician.

Nonprescription sleep aids

A variety of over-the-counter agents is available, each of which claims to combat sleepless nights. Americans spend several hundred million dollars per year on nonprescription sleep aids. Many of these products contain antihistamines and herbs. More significant is that the U.S. Food and Drug Administration does not regulate the safety, efficacy, or purity of these preparations. As such, none of them have been studied thoroughly. Some patients do feel that antihistamines help them sleep better, but this effect has not been demonstrated in research studies. Antihistamines may improve short-term insomnia to some extent, but side effects often outweigh their benefits.

Melatonin: Melatonin is one of the most popular nonprescription sleep aids. A naturally occurring hormone, melatonin is secreted in the brain by the pineal gland to promote sleep. Levels of this hormone increase in the brain shortly after darkness, peak between 2 A.M. and 4 A.M., and then decrease gradually in the morning. Melatonin has been demonstrated to be effective in treating sleep problems that accompany jet lag and night shift rescheduling, but its benefits for insomnia are much more variable. Over-the-counter melatonin is extracted from animals, hence the purity of the preparation cannot always be guaranteed. Dizziness, headaches, fatigue, and irritability are common side effects.

Antihistamines: Antihistamines are the major ingredient in many nonprescription sleep aids. Three antihistamines—diphenhydramine hydrochloride, diphenhydramine citrate, and doxylamine succinate—are currently approved by the FDA for this purpose.

FDA Issues Warning on Sleeping Pills

In 2007, the Food and Drug Administration mandated that manufacturers of sedative-hypnotic drugs strengthen their product labeling to include stronger language to describe the potential risks associated with using the drugs. These risks include severe allergic reactions, severe facial swelling, memory lapses, hallucinations, and complex sleep-related behaviors. The behaviors occur with no recollection whatsoever, after a person takes a pill and heads for bed. Drinking alcohol around the same time as taking these drugs increases the chances of having such a reaction. Some of the behaviors reported by sleeping pill consumers include:

- Sleep-driving
- Making phone calls while asleep
- Making internet purchases asleep
- Preparing and eating food while asleep
- Engaging in sexual activities while asleep

Side effects include residual daytime sedation, diminished cognitive function, and delirium, the latter being more common in the elderly. Others include dry mouth, blurred vision, urinary retention, constipation, and risk of increased intraocular pressure in individuals with glaucoma. Antihistamines have not been rigorously studied for insomnia and safety and efficacy data are limited.

Alcohol: Many people with insomnia use alcohol to fall asleep. In fact, alcohol is often the first thing an insomniac will try. Although alcohol can help a person fall asleep, it is also associated with poor sleep quality and night awakenings. The routine use of alcohol as a sleep aid can lead to abuse, tolerance, and dependence and is strongly discouraged.

Alternative therapies

A number of herbal supplements are thought to be effective in the treatment of insomnia. However none of these therapies have undergone rigorous scrutiny and published work on herbal hypnotics is limited. Examples include kava, valerian, lavender, chamomile, and ylang-ylang. Reports of liver failure associated with kava led to it being banned in parts of Europe in 2002. In 2005, the Food and Drug Administration issued an advisory regarding the potential risk for serious liver injury.

See Appendix 3 for a list of commonly used over-the-counter sleep aids.

Chapter 9

Sleep Terrors

Sleep is when all the unsorted stuff comes flying out as from a dustbin upset in a high wind.
—William Golding

Sleep terrors are characterized by a sudden arousal from slow wave sleep. The sleeper will scream, cry, sit up, sweat, have a rapid heartbeat, and display a look of fear. Patients most often do not remember these episodes, which occur most often during sleep stage 3.

Caleb

Caleb's blood-curdling scream jarred his mother from a deep sleep. She ran down the hall, threw open the door to her 7-year-old son's bedroom, and found him sitting upright in his bed—eyes wide open, breathing like he'd been playing tag, rocking back and forth and mumbling incoherently.

"Caleb, wake up! It's okay—I'm here."

Caleb looked through his mother as though she were a ghost. The eerie disconnect worried Sandy. She had been certain that after tucking him into bed more than an hour ago, he would sleep through the night this time. She held Caleb's trembling body close to her while he cried, and she smoothed his crop of tousled hair. Caleb carried on for at least five minutes.

Caleb's episodes are happening more frequently. The previous week, he woke up almost every night—always about an hour after going to bed. The episodes worry Sandy because Caleb never remembers the horrible incidents that scare him into a panic each night. Sometimes he is aggressive, thrashing and protesting when Sandy tries to shake him out of his frightened stupor. Just recently, he ran out of his bedroom, down the stairs, and toward the front door. Fortunately, the door was locked. Despite her efforts, Sandy's attempts to calm him down are futile.

Sandy called Caleb's pediatrician to discuss the behavior, and both agreed that Caleb is not simply having recurring bad dreams. Caleb's behavior worries the doctor. The young boy could accidentally hurt himself or someone else. The doctor suggested that Caleb and his mother see a sleep specialist.

Caleb's Sleep Assessment

Sleep snapshot

Caleb's bedtime is between 8:30 and 9 P.M., and he slept soundly through the night before his incidents began a few months ago. His frightening episodes usually occur in cycles, eventually increasing in frequency to every night for a week and then disappearing for months on end. He does not display excessive daytime sleepiness or difficulty falling back asleep after one of his episodes.

The sleep specialist recommended an overnight sleep study for Caleb, but told Sandy that he suspected sleep terrors. He felt a polysomnogram would rule out disorders known to aggravate sleep terrors, such as sleep apnea, since Sandy reported that Caleb occasionally snores. A polysomnogram might differentiate sleep terrors from nocturnal seizures, a condition also characterized by recurrent episodes of abnormal behaviors in sleep. Because Caleb is quite young, his mother was asked to accompany him to the lab and stay with him during the study.

During the study, Caleb did not present with typical symptoms of disorders such as restless legs syndrome or apnea, nor did the test results indicate cause for serious concern about nocturnal seizures. Caleb's physician advised Sandy to videotape Caleb while he slept at home so she could capture an episode for closer examination.

In cases like Caleb's a videotape may play a critical role in generating a diagnosis, and conducting a "study" at home may be as effective as checking into a lab. Your doctor will advise if this is a viable option. Sandy captured several of Caleb's episodes on tape, and the physician observed the recordings. The similarity of one event to another—in terms of the time the event occurred, the time between Caleb's bedtime and the onset of the event, and his facial expressions and vocalizations during the event—helped Caleb's physician make a diagnosis.

Excessive daytime sleepiness

Despite nightly interruptions in his sleep, Caleb does not exhibit signs of daytime sleepiness. He does not nap during the day and appears to be a happy, even-tempered child.

Medical and family history

In general, Caleb is a healthy boy, and his medical records show no medical or psychological concerns.

The diagnosis

After reviewing the videotapes, the sleep specialist diagnosed Caleb with sleep terrors. Caleb's behavior aligned with the disorder's symptoms: abrupt arousal from deep sleep, screaming, crying, pallor, panic, and lack of response to attempts to wake him.

All about Sleep Terrors

Sleep terrors are a mysterious sleep disorder in the parasomnia category in which patients experience an incomplete arousal from deep sleep. The patient appears to be aware but is usually unresponsive to the environment and typically has no memory of what transpired the next morning. Sleep terrors tend to happen in cycles; a person may experience one episode in his or her entire life or recurrent episodes as often as every night.

Who gets sleep terrors?

Sleep terrors are most common in children between the ages of 3 and 12, and they tend to resolve during adolescence. As many as 6 percent of children may experience sleep terrors. A much smaller population of adults—closer to 2 percent—experience this disorder. If they occur in adulthood, incidents are most common between the ages of 20 and 30. Few individuals over age 65 experience sleep terrors. Family history may play a strong role in whether your child will experience these episodes.

Sleep terrors often occur or increase in frequency during times of stress or exhaustion. A child who is going through a transition in school or had an exhausting day is more likely to experience an episode.

How do I know if I have sleep terrors?

People who have sleep terrors usually do not remember the incidents. Rarely, the patient may recall portions of a vivid dream that was frightening in nature. In fact, when an observer watches a patient experience a sleep terror, the patient looks truly frightened. During the terror, the patient's eyes may open, pupils dilate, and he or she may sit up in bed abruptly and breathe heavily. Heart rate during these incidents can pump up to 200 beats per minute, far exceeding the normal, resting heart rate. The episode might last between

5 and 20 minutes, during which time the person might scream out, babble incoherently, thrash, and in some cases, bolt out of bed and run out of the room. (The latter is more common in adults.)

Adults who live alone and suffer from sleep terrors and related disorders typically are not aware of their nighttime activities unless they awaken during the episode or leave behind evidence of mishap. Patients may awaken to find themselves sitting on the side of the bed or standing in another room if the episode involved sleepwalking. Rarely, parasomnia sufferers wake up to find their bedcovers a mess and the contents of the bedside table on the floor.

Sleep terrors are potentially dangerous. Patients who suffer from them can injure themselves unknowingly. Patients are difficult to arouse during sleep terrors, and they may be confused or disoriented upon awakening. Because the majority of stage 3 sleep occurs in the first third of the sleep period, episodes also tend to occur during this time.

When disturbed sleepers do remember sleep terror incidents, they often report seeing animals—often snakes or spiders—or people. Science cannot explain this imagery.

Many individuals who suffer from sleep terrors are misdiagnosed. Children are often told, "It's just a nightmare, don't worry." Adults, on the other hand, may be misdiagnosed with post-traumatic stress disorder or nocturnal panic disorder. It is important to understand the distinctions among these disorders and to note that sleep terrors are a frightening, confusing experience for sleepers and observers alike. You can't shake a person out of a sleep terror, and the frightened sleeper will not respond to your voice no matter how loudly you speak. The best thing to do is to stand nearby and make sure the person is not injured during the episode. Of course, this might not be possible if the person is thrashing or violent, which is more common in adults. Attempts to restrain the sleeper may provoke more aggressive responses.

An overnight sleep study can help determine which stage of sleep the patient is in when the terror occurs. If increased brain activity is detected during slow wave sleep, then a diagnosis of sleep terrors is likely. However, in many cases, sleep terrors can be diagnosed by the sleep history alone.

Nightmare or sleep terror? Nightmares are frightening dreams that typically cause awakenings from sleep. Nightmares generally begin between 3 and 6 years of age and can scare young children so much that they may be afraid to go back to sleep. As many as 50 percent of children at this age have nightmares that are significant enough to disturb their sleep, and therefore, their parents' sleep. Like sleep terrors, nightmares decrease in frequency as children age.

One key differentiation between a sleep terror and a nightmare is the time of the episode. Because sleep terrors occur during deep sleep, episodes take place during the first part of the night, usually an hour or two after bedtime. On the other hand, nightmares, which usually occur during rapid eye movement sleep, occur toward the end of the night. But there are exceptions to this rule.

Another distinction between a sleep terror and a nightmare is whether you can wake the person during the episode. During a sleep terror, a person's eyes may open, but he or she will see right

Nightmares versus Sleep Terrors

Not sure if your child—or spouse—is waking up frightened from a sleep terror or nightmare? Here is the difference:

Sleep Terror	Nightmare
Occurs during the first third of night	Occurs during REM sleep (usually last third of night)
Will not respond to touch	Will respond to touch and comforting sound, or attempts to comfort
Confused after episode; doesn't remember episode	Is fully awake after episode; often recalls dreams

through you. In fact, the sleeper has no idea you are present and will not respond to your voice or touch. If, on the other hand, the incident is a nightmare, the person's eyes may open and he or she may scream, but the frightened individual usually awakens because of the dream and will respond to comforting.

What causes sleep terrors?

People afflicted with sleep terrors, confusional arousals, and sleep-walking are believed to have abnormal arousal mechanisms in slow-wave sleep. This results in partial arousals from deep NREM sleep during which the patient typically has little or no memory. Genetic factors play a major role. More than 80 percent of people with sleepwalking or sleep terrors have relatives who suffer with similar problems. The chances a child will develop sleep terrors or a related disorder increase if a parent is affected by the disorder; the chances are even higher if both parents are affected. In a minority of cases, factors other than genetics, such as stress or medications, are implicated.

Some triggers for sleep terrors, sleepwalking, and confusional arousals include:

- lack of sleep
- interrupted sleep or inefficient sleep (including from shift work, sleep apnea, and limb movements in sleep)
- illness or fever
- certain medications, drugs, and alcohol
- stress
- going to bed with a full bladder
- noisy sleep environment/different sleep environment
- psychiatric disorders (including bipolar disorder, depression, and anxiety)

During stage 3 of NREM sleep, the brain is in its deepest state of rest—a state in which both the mind and body rejuvenate. Arousing from deep sleep is not the norm. Unlike during REM sleep, when the body is essentially paralyzed, a person's body will react during the periods of time when brain activity transitions into sleep. This usually occurs within the first hour after sleep onset. The person is still sleeping but able to act out. Bed-wetting, sleep-talking, and sleepwalking also occur during stage 3 sleep.

The Polysomnogram

To prepare Caleb for his polysomnogram, technologists applied electrodes to Caleb's scalp and attached other sensors to record his breathing, heart rate, oxygen level, and body movements while he slept. Prior to the study, his mother signed a consent form for Caleb to be videotaped. (Routine during overnight sleep studies, videotaping allows physicians to correlate brain and breathing signals with movements and behaviors in sleep.)

Not surprisingly, the young boy did not have any abnormal activity through the night, other than some difficulty in falling asleep due to the sensors and the strange environment. The negative polysomnogram did not confirm the suspected diagnosis, but it did rule out other sleep disorders, such as periodic limb movements and apnea. It also allowed Caleb's physician to rule out epileptic seizures. Negative polysomnograms in this setting are not uncommon, the physician explained to Caleb's mother. The best way to diagnose Caleb's sleep problem was for his mother to videotape him sleeping at home in his own bed.

How to Get a Good Night's Sleep

Parents should not try to yell, coax, or shake a child out of a sleep terror, sleepwalking episode, or a confusional arousal. During this deep sleep stage, the child is having an incomplete arousal; this means he or she is still technically asleep, yet able to move and appearing awake. Your child likely will not remember the incident, so pressing for information or explanations the next morning will only produce frustration. Instead, if you notice that sleep terrors are a pattern, stand at the bedroom doorway and observe your child. Call your pediatrician and explain the behavior.

General measures

Most arousal disorders do not require medical treatment. Sleepers suffering from a sleep terror, especially young children, may unknowingly appreciate a hug and comforting touch. Although they will probably not respond to comforting actions, holding a child is a natural and healthy reaction to sleep terrors. A different course of action must be taken with adults who suffer from sleep terrors because they are more likely to manifest aggressive behavior or thrashing, which can injure anyone attempting to comfort them. In these cases, it's best to stand back and let the terror run its course. For children with frequent sleep terrors, some sleep experts recommend gently waking a child shortly before the usual time of an episode, a technique known as anticipatory awakening. This will disrupt the child's sleep cycle and reduce the chance a terror will occur. However, this could also cause your child to lose more sleep without actually affecting behavior as he or she progresses into deeper sleep stages.

Because exhaustion and stress can spur sleep terrors, parents must ensure that their child gets enough rest. If your child usually takes a nap, make sure there is time set aside each day for this important period of rest. If bedtimes are getting later and wake-up calls earlier, adjust sleep schedules so your child won't wear out during the day. Normal routines foster healthy sleep habits, and your child's activities during the day will impact his or her ability to sleep soundly. Make sure the hour before bedtime is quiet and relaxing. Avoid television, computer games, and scary bedtime stories. Report all sleep problems to your child's doctor. If there is an underlying disorder like sleep apnea or periodic limb movements, the sleep terrors may be resolved if the underlying disorder is treated.

Follow these tips to ensure your child's safety during the night:

- Secure all doors and windows in the house to prevent the sleepwalker from escaping unnoticed.

- Clear your child's bedroom of clutter and pad furniture to avoid injury.

- Place gates at all stairways.

- Use bells or another alerting device on your child's bedroom door and windows so others in the house will be alerted if an episode occurs.

- If you find your child sleepwalking, gently coax him or her back to bed. Never shake your child awake. This may provoke confusion and violent, aggressive behavior.

Medication

Certain medications may be prescribed to calm sleep terrors. These are used as a temporary solution. Owing to the frequency and severity of his sleep terrors, Caleb was prescribed imipramine, which also is used to treat bed-wetting. Other possible medications include diazepam and amitryptiline. Medications are generally reserved for severe cases when episodes occur frequently or are particularly disruptive to others in the household, lead to daytime difficulties for the patient, or pose a risk of injury. Your doctor will indicate whether medication is appropriate.

Caleb's Outcome

Caleb was treated with imipramine, which significantly reduced the frequency and severity of the episodes. After 18 months of treatment, his physician gradually withdrew the medication and he remained spell-free.

Chapter 10

Rapid Eye Movement Behavior Disorder

If you want your spouse to listen and pay strict attention to every word you say, talk in your sleep.

—Anonymous

REM behavior disorder occurs when the physical paralysis characteristic of REM sleep is incomplete or absent. This condition allows individuals to act out their dreams.

Janet and Tom

Janet and Tom never pick fights with one another. Their happy, 15-year marriage has been punctuated by only a few real arguments. Tom simply isn't a confrontational person, and Janet would rather compromise than bicker. Lately, however, Tom's behavior has changed—but only while he sleeps.

Janet regularly wakes up to a kicking, thrashing, seemingly angry Tom. He flails his arms, slamming his fist on the mattress like a gavel while he speaks loudly, often swearing.

Tom never talked like that in the past. He always kept his cool, no matter how angry he was.

When he wakes, Tom doesn't remember the confrontations, no matter how violent or disturbing they were. He has always had vivid dreams and, though he admits he sometimes can't separate reveries from reality during sleep, the actual content of his recent nighttime outbursts surprises him. Janet worries he will hurt himself—or her. She connects his vulgar and angry language to past arguments with subordinates at work. Tom, 62, was diagnosed with Parkinson's disease eight years ago and retired four years ago.

In addition to his recent sleep disturbances, Tom is more forgetful and struggles to concentrate. He complains that his restless nights take a toll on his energy level. He wakes up between four and six times each night and does not fall back asleep easily. He snores, suffers from daytime sleepiness, and can't restrain his nocturnal activities. What's more, his condition seems to be worsening. Recently, he gave Janet a black eye during a nocturnal struggle.

Tom's Sleep Assessment

Sleep snapshot

Tom turns in at 9 P.M. and awakens at 5 A.M. He says six hours of sleep is sufficient, but he generally gets only four to five hours of rest each night, interrupted by frequent awakenings.

Excessive daytime sleepiness

Tom wakes up refreshed in the morning, but he always takes early evening naps. By then, his sleepless night catches up with him, and he feels much better if he can capture 10 to 20 minutes of shut-eye before dinner. Tom denies excessive daytime sleepiness, but the physician scored Tom's Epworth Sleepiness Scale at 15 out of 24—a rating that is significantly higher than normal.

Medical and family history

Tom was diagnosed with Parkinson's disease after he developed a hand tremor, which was followed a few years later by gait difficulties and memory trouble. He takes levodopa to control the tremor, but his motor and cognitive problems have persisted and were responsible for his early retirement. His father's sister, now deceased, had Alzheimer's disease. His father died in his 50s following a heart attack. Tom has two younger sisters who are healthy, although one was recently diagnosed with RLS.

Parasomnias Tom's behavior is characteristic of a parasomnia, a disorder in which the patient experiences unusual sleep behavior, often without recollection. These disorders usually arise during NREM sleep. During these periods of apparent wakefulness, patients engage in unusual behavior such as sleepwalking, sleep-talking, or sleep-related eating.

Tom acts out his dreams. His episodes almost always occur in the early morning hours, and he sometimes recalls vivid, frightening dreams where he feels he is threatened or chased. These symptoms suggest the problem may be occurring during REM sleep. During this stage, the body is paralyzed, but the mind is active. A normal sleeper's still body isn't in sync with his or her active brain, which prevents the sleeper from acting out dreams. In Tom's case, his body is not paralyzed in REM sleep as it should be, allowing him to move in response to threatening dreams.

The diagnosis

Tom displays symptoms of REM behavior disorder (RBD), when paralysis that should occur during REM is cut short or not present at all. He dreams wildly and has the ability to act out each scene.

Parkinson's disease is known to be associated with RBD. In fact, 80 percent of patients with this neurodegenerative disorder also suffer from a primary sleep disorder. Tom's violent bedtime behavior has worsened since he was diagnosed with Parkinson's disease, but Janet remembers Tom having occasional screaming spells years before the Parkinson's set in.

After conducting a sleep interview with Tom, RBD was an obvious conclusion. The physician ordered an overnight polysomnogram with expanded EMG and EEG sensors to collect more detailed brain-wave and muscle activity data. Additional sensors help confirm an RBD diagnosis by analyzing the level of muscle activity during REM sleep. Expanded information is critical to ruling out the multitude of other sleep disorders known to affect Parkinson's patients, including restless legs syndrome, periodic limb movement disorder, sleep apnea, and daytime sleepiness spurred by medications.

All about REM Behavior Disorder

Some of the most unusual sleep stories come from individuals with REM behavior disorder. Edward, a World War II veteran, broke his foot kicking a bedpost he mistook for the enemy. Another patient was locked into his bedroom each night by his wife because his behavior was so disturbing and violent. Still another dreamed he was being chased, punching his wife in the ribcage unknowingly in the process of trying to get away. One restless sleeper, an otherwise kind man, took a swing at his mate when he dreamed he was in the middle of a standoff.

Most RBD patients are, in fact, men. A typical profile is a male over age 60 who might demonstrate other brain disorders. RBD is not a psychiatric disorder, but it is a potentially dangerous neurological condition. The good news is that the disorder can be treated.

The REM behavior disorder falls into the REM parasomnia category. There are a dozen parasomnias, and they can occur in both REM and NREM sleep stages. Most common are sleep-talking and sleepwalking. But RBD takes parasomnias to a new level. Rather than strolling around like a zombie, individuals afflicted with RBD are animated and involved in their dreams.

Because it occurs during REM sleep, when the body is supposed to be paralyzed, RBD is differentiated from arousal disorders. During episodes of RBD there is loss of REM sleep atonia—the limp, paralyzed state associated with this sleep stage—which allows those with the disorder to move freely, even violently. Kicking, thrashing, and swinging—in an attempt to escape from someone or something chasing them—are not unusual actions for RBD patients.

Incidents typically occur in the last one-third of the sleep period, when REM sleep predominates. But they can occur as early as 90 minutes after sleep onset during the first REM period. Violent episodes can occur as infrequently as a few times in a lifetime or as frequently as several times over several consecutive nights. Most patients complain of sleep injury but rarely cite sleep disruption, as they usually do not wake up until a family member jerks them back into reality. Once awake, patients often recall their dramatic dreams.

Who gets RBD?

The disorder usually surfaces in men aged 50 or older. It is linked to medical problems, most notably Parkinson's disease and related neurodegenerative disorders associated with dementia, strokes, and narcolepsy. In fact, 30 percent of Parkinson's patients have RBD, and symptoms of RBD may precede other neurological problems by up to ten years. Three-quarters of men who have RBD may eventually develop degenerative disorders similar to Parkinson's disease. In some instances, a temporary form of RBD can occur during withdrawal from alcohol, sedatives, or some antidepressants.

How do I know I have RBD?

Patients who have the disorder may display one or more of the following symptoms. Ask yourself these questions:

- Do you act out dreams?

- Do you ever thrash, punch, kick, or use vulgar language during sleep, and do you recall these incidents?

- Do you recall vivid, threatening dreams after waking?

- Are you tired during the day because of restless nights?

- Does your bed partner complain of violent behavior or does your partner notice activity while you sleep?

There are several levels of RBD. Mild cases display behavior less than once per month and cause mild discomfort to bed partners. Patients with moderate RBD act out less than once a week and create a physically uncomfortable situation for their bed partners. Patients with severe RBD are violent and cause physical injury to themselves and their bed partners.

What causes RBD?

Onset of REM behavior disorder occurs when specific parts of the brain that interrupt muscle paralysis in REM sleep and disinhibit motor pathways are disturbed. Disorders of neurodegeneration, including Parkinson's disease, dementia with Lewy bodies, and multiple system atrophy, are the leading triggers for RBD. The disorder occurs more commonly in patients with narcolepsy and other neurological disorders, including multiple sclerosis, stroke, and brain tumors. Alcohol withdrawal can trigger an acute form of RBD. Certain medications, particularly venlafaxine, and other antidepressants in the selective serotonin reuptake inhibitor and tricyclic antidepressant classes can also trigger RBD attacks.

RBD and neurodegenerative diseases There is an increased rate of RBD in people with neurodegenerative diseases, and the latest research suggests that RBD could be a sign of other degenerative processes in the central nervous system.

If RBD is one of the earliest stages on the neurodegenerative spectrum, perhaps in the future, physicians could test for RBD and treat patients with medication that may ward off these more debilitating disorders. Researchers are hopeful that medical advances will make earlier identification and treatment possible in years to come.

The Polysomnogram

During REM sleep, patients with REM behavior disorder will show signs of augmented muscle tone. If awakened during an episode, a patient might relay a dream that correlates with his or her physical activity. Periodic leg movements, arm activity, and otherwise restless behavior are also observed in sleepers diagnosed with RBD.

How to Get a Good Night's Sleep

Sleep histories are critical in making an RBD diagnosis. A polysomnogram helps to confirm the diagnosis and rule out other sleep disorders, such as periodic limb movements and sleep apnea. A physician might order other tests, such as brain imaging, to determine whether a patient has associated neurological disorders as well.

Medication

Typically, REM behavior disorder can be treated with medications used to suppress REM sleep, which also inhibits physical activity. Clonazepam, a drug in the benzodiazepine class, is the most common medication used to treat RBD and is effective in 90 percent of cases. Other drugs that may reduce RBD episodes include melatonin and dopamine agonists, such as pramipexole, which is used to treat Parkinson's disease and restless legs syndrome. Safety measures should be implemented to reduce the risk of injury to the patient and his or her bed partner. Removing bedside furniture and adding padding to nearby walls or furniture is recommended. In some cases, securing a safe environment includes moving the bed partner into another room. This is a particularly important step because RBD patients are known for mistaking their spouse for an aggressor and acting out forcefully in self-defense.

Tom's Outcome

In addition to the polysomnogram showing nearly continuous limb (leg and arm) movements during both NREM and REM sleep, Tom displayed periodic leg movements when he was awake at the start of the study. During NREM sleep, particularly during stages 1 and 2, frequent periodic limb movements caused arousal, leading to excessive fragmentation of sleep. In REM sleep, he showed elevated amounts of muscle tone in his arms and legs, and had a couple of episodes where he vocalized incoherently and flailed his arms, but nothing as dramatic as the episodes he has experienced at home.

Tom was placed on clonazepam, a drug in the benzodiazepine class, which is considered a sedative hypnotic. This is the treatment of choice for RBD, and even low doses are able to abolish spells as it did for Tom and does in most cases. This agent is also effective in treating restless legs syndrome and periodic limb movement disorder.

Chapter 11

Circadian Rhythm Sleep Disorders

Delayed Sleep-Phase Syndrome

"Dawn: when men of reason go to bed."
—Ambrose Bierce

Circadian rhythm sleep disorders occur when normal sleep-wake rhythms are disturbed, often when an individual's natural sleep-wake schedule does not conform to society's norm. These disorders are caused by alterations of the internal body clock or misalignment between the body's internal rhythms and environmental factors.

Delayed sleep-phase syndrome is a circadian rhythm disorder most common in adolescents and young adults, whose night owl tendencies delay sleep onset—often until 2 A.M. or later. Early wake times result in sleep-deprivation, daytime sleepiness, and impaired work and school performance.

Andy never was a morning person. He hits his peak at 10 P.M. and can't fall asleep until after 2 A.M., no matter how hard he tries. Even when he was in high school, when his mother turned off the television promptly at 10 P.M., he would lie in bed wide-awake until well after midnight. She always figured Andy was asleep, and she never understood why he was so groggy at breakfast.

When Andy, now 20, went away to college, the late-night/party weekend schedule of the typical freshman year jibed with his own night-owl tendencies. He routinely turned out the lights at 1 A.M. during the week. But Andy's internal closing time on Friday and Saturday nights (and sometimes on Thursdays as well, if Friday classes were canceled) usually neared 3 or 4 A.M. He slept away Saturday and Sunday mornings, waking barely in time for lunch.

Andy attributed his routine to campus life. When his mother expressed concern, he shrugged, rolled his eyes, and said, "Whatever, Mom."

Now Andy is a sophomore, and he's no longer able to avoid early morning classes. On two mornings each week, he has lab at 9 A.M., and on the other three mornings, he's faced with a history class at 8 A.M. Despite the shift in his schedule, Andy can't seem to adjust his bedtime to get the sleep he needs. He's tried everything: reading, avoiding weekday activities, and even taking over-the-counter sleep aids. Nothing works. Alcohol makes him feel less rested the next day.

Now, Andy's grades are slipping. And his mother is asking questions.

Andy's Sleep Assessment

Sleep snapshot

Andy doesn't fall asleep until 1 or 2 A.M. during the week, and he maintains a much later bedtime on weekends. On a positive note, however, is the fact that although Andy has been unable to alter his bedtime—he lies in bed awake when he tries—it is consistent. Once Andy falls asleep, he sleeps soundly until morning (or early afternoon). He usually sleeps for six hours each night. On weekends, when he can sleep late, he gets a solid eight hours, sometimes ten hours, and often feels great when he wakes up. He's sluggish primarily during the school week, when he is forced to rise earlier than he would like.

Excessive daytime sleepiness

Andy isn't alert in the morning, and he drags through afternoons because he is so tired from waking up for early classes. Because campus life is so busy, he rarely has time for naps. But he has been observed snoozing in Chemistry 101—the professor made him aware of that.

Andy's teachers have pointed out his slipping grades. He's a bright, creative student, but his professors don't see him performing at his peak; they only know the tired, unmotivated slacker.

Insomnia

Because Andy struggles to fall asleep at night, his mother questioned whether his delayed sleep onset was a sign of insomnia. Andy is also worried, and he wondered if he was narcoleptic because he falls asleep during class and has even nodded off while driving.

Medical and family history

Andy's mother finds his behavior unusual. She and her husband both sleep soundly, with the exception of some occasional snoring. In fact, her sleep routine is quite the opposite of Andy's, and she usually awakens in a cheerful frame of mind, chirping "good morning" to her grouchy son. Neither she nor her husband have been diagnosed or treated for sleep disorders.

The diagnosis

Andy's physician requested that he keep a sleep diary for two weeks, recording the following information:

- Bedtime and wake time
- How long it took to fall asleep
- Number of awakenings during the night; length of these awakenings
- Number of times he got out of bed
- Total sleep time
- How he felt when he woke up in the morning
- Number and quality of daytime naps

A tailored test for Andy Andy maintained a sleep log and wore an actigraph, a wristwatch-like device that measured his activity level day and night during the two weeks. With the data in hand, the

Tailored Tests

Tailoring sleep lab tests is critical to properly diagnosing many sleep disorders. If Andy, for example, had not kept a sleep diary or provided a sleep history, the physician would not know that the young man habitually falls asleep at 2 A.M., rarely wakes up, and can sleep soundly for hours if allowed. This information is critical to tailoring the sleep study to diagnose Andy's problem. Daytime tests typically begin around 8 A.M. Had Andy been awakened by the technician to start the daytime test at the standard time, the results might have led to a misdiagnosis. Andy might have appeared to have insomnia or difficulty adjusting to the sleep lab environment. During his MSLT, his sleep latency might have been only minutes, and he might have plunged into REM sleep, which would have suggested narcolepsy.

Neither of these diagnoses would have been accurate for Andy.

physician noticed an obvious sleep pattern: Andy's sleep differed dramatically on weekdays compared to weekends. On weekends, he slept soundly for eight to ten hours, and he usually woke refreshed if he didn't have to get up early. But his bedtimes and wake times on weekends were out of sync with what most people consider normal.

The physician ordered an overnight sleep study and MSLT so he could observe Andy's sleep-wake cycle in the lab. Because the physician already understood Andy's sleep patterns, the polysomnogram and MSLT were tailored to meet his habits. That way, the study would produce the best results because it would measure Andy's cycles when his body naturally triggered sleep.

All about Delayed Sleep Phase Syndrome

Individuals with Delayed Sleep Phase Syndrome (DSPS) struggle to wake up for work or school and find themselves lying awake at night, trying to force themselves to fall asleep before their bodies are ready. They often are chronically tardy or perform poorly on the job. But you can't force people with DSPS to fall asleep, and you can't shift their circadian rhythm without proper treatment.

Because those diagnosed with DSPS suffer from sleep deprivation, many of them turn to caffeinated or energy drinks in an effort to stay awake. Many may resort to over-the-counter stimulants. To sleep at night, people who suffer from DSPS often try sleep aids, but most of them find the pills rarely have an effect. Some sufferers turn to alcohol, but this serves only to worsen their sleep cycles, perpetuate symptoms, and, in some cases, lead to substance abuse.

Who gets DSPS?

Delayed sleep phase syndrome (DSPS) often surfaces during adolescent and early adult years. Patients diagnosed with the disorder have difficulty conforming to society's time schedule and often are perceived as lazy, unmotivated, or poor performers.

In fact, people like Andy are productive, alert, and creative later at night. The problem is a conflict between these individuals' circadian rhythms and what is expected or considered the norm.

College life mimics the schedules that are normal to people who suffer from DSPS. Young adults may adopt poor sleep hygiene while they are in college and, as a result, develop alternative sleeping patterns. They stay up late, sleep in late, and make up for lost sleep on weekends. Sleeping for eight hours isn't a problem—as long as it's on their schedules.

Unfortunately, when these individuals graduate and move into standard employment settings, they are forced to conform to the schedules set by their employers, which inevitably leads to sleep deprivation and, ultimately, problems with performance and behavior during the day.

How do I know I have DSPS?

The following are common symptoms of delayed sleep phase syndrome:

- Sleep onset is later than desired, usually between 1 and 6 A.M., but occurs at the same time each night
- Wake times in the late morning or early afternoon if the sleeper is left undisturbed
- Little or no difficulty staying asleep following sleep onset
- Difficulty waking in the early morning
- Inability to fall asleep earlier
- Daytime sleepiness, resulting in unplanned naps and feeling unrefreshed after waking
- Poor academic performance, falling asleep during classes or being unproductive at work, a reputation for being lazy or unmotivated, and chronically tardy for morning activities

What causes DSPS?

Approximately 7 to 16 percent of adolescents and young adults are affected by DSPS, but the cause of the condition remains poorly understood. Several factors may contribute to the onset of delayed sleep phase syndrome. Some scientists think DSPS may be an exaggerated reaction to the normal scheduling shift that takes place in the body's internal clocks after puberty. Other researchers have discovered derangements in a circadian clock gene in patients with DSPS, which may be responsible for triggering symptom onset. Environmental factors, such as reduced light exposure in the morning, excessive bright light exposure in the evening, shift work, and traveling across time zones, can also precipitate the disorder.

The Polysomnogram

Because of Andy's tendency to stay awake at night and sleep late in the morning, a tailored polysomnogram was important to diagnose Andy's sleep problem. In the lab, Andy fell asleep around 3 A.M., which was matched what his physician expected he would do. His polysomnogram showed a few arousals during sleep, but no significant apnea episodes or limb movements. Because technicians knew about Andy's established sleep patterns, they allowed him to sleep much later than the typical 6 A.M. wake-up time so they could record his complete sleep period. He slept for nearly eight hours.

Andy's MSLT started at noon rather than at 8 A.M., when the test is typically administered. His sleep latency during the MSLT was nine minutes, and he did not enter REM sleep. He described his sleep in the lab as typical for a weekend.

Andy's results ruled out insomnia and narcolepsy. He did not nap frequently or have any of the other cardinal features of narcolepsy. The physician knew that Andy's sleep onset was delayed during the polysomnogram because his circadian clock was timed so he wants to sleep much later than the average person. Unlike insomniacs,

Andy did not experience frequent arousals or stay awake for long periods of time during the night, nor did he have anxiety about not being able to fall asleep at night. Although he didn't fall asleep until 3 A.M., the delayed onset was typical behavior according to his sleep log.

Based on this information, the physician diagnosed Andy with delayed sleep phase syndrome.

How to Get a Good Night's Sleep

The best ways to treat DSPS are to employ tactics that promote earlier sleep and wake-up times. Practicing good sleep hygiene (discussed in chapter 8) is the first step toward creating a relaxing, sleep-promoting environment, but there are also other ways to adjust circadian rhythm.

Essentially, patients with delayed sleep phase syndrome need to trick their biological clocks into thinking it is time for bed between 10 P.M. and midnight, and they need to promote wakefulness at an hour that is more socially acceptable, such as 7 A.M. To do this, a physician might prescribe melatonin or suggest light therapy.

Therapy

Light therapy Daylight signals the body it's time to wake up. Consistent exposure to bright light tends to lead to earlier wake-up times and to advance sleep onset at night. Patients can receive this therapy at home by using a light box, which emits a high dosage of light quantified in a unit known as *lux* (a measurement of illumination). The light's brightness mirrors natural sunlight. A DSPS sleeper is instructed to clip the light to his or her bed, position it at a specified distance from the face, and turn it on in the morning after waking. The lights also can be put on a timer, which improves compliance for most DSPS patients, who are just as likely to avoid the bright light as a buzzing alarm clock. The light stimulates the brain to wake up even if the patient is lying in bed with eyes closed.

Dosage and timing of light treatment is tailored to the patient. For some, light exposure beginning at 7 A.M. may gradually advance sleep onset at night by a couple of hours. In addition to using the light in the morning, it's equally important for the person with DSPS to avoid bright light exposure in the evening. Sufferers should minimize time spent in brightly lit rooms, in front of computer screens, or under other sources of light after 8 P.M.

Medication

Melatonin You may have heard of melatonin as a remedy for jet lag. Melatonin is a hormone normally secreted by the pineal gland in the brain to promote sleep. Melatonin excretion occurs when it is dark; daylight suppresses melatonin. In people with DSPS, melatonin release may be delayed, which explains why they may not feel sleepy until the early morning hours. Melatonin levels can be checked to confirm the diagnosis, but this is usually done for research purposes. To jump-start the brain's natural melatonin secretion, a physician may prescribe a specific dosage of melatonin to be taken several hours before bedtime (6 P.M. is a good starting point for many patients).

Andy's Outcome

At first, Andy's case sounds like a typical transition to college life, but the truth is that Andy was facing a serious sleep deficit that affected his mood and performance in school—and, ultimately, his future. To gradually shift Andy's bedtime to midnight, the physician prescribed melatonin in addition to morning light therapy. Andy found the treatment tedious at first but changed his attitude as his performance improved.

At school, Andy's no longer dragged himself out of bed to get to class, and he stopped dozing in sedentary situations. His grades and his attention span during class improved. Andy maintained the same treatment on weekends to develop a consistent schedule. He accepted that DSPS is a lifelong condition, and he felt at ease knowing that treatment would help him achieve his goals and keep up with his friends and colleagues.

Other Circadian Rhythm Disorders

Delayed sleep phase syndrome is the most common circadian rhythm disorder among adolescents and young adults, but other populations also experience sleep deprivation from a skewed body clock. Do your sleep patterns match society's ideas of appropriate bedtimes and wake-up calls?

Following are a few disorders that occur when lifestyle plays with sleep cycles:

Advanced sleep phase syndrome

The opposite of DSPS, ASPS is most common in mature adults, who naturally want to go to bed earlier. A senior citizen may fall asleep at 6 P.M. and wake up at 2 A.M. This pattern can disrupt social activities during the day because the individual is fatigued from such an uncommonly early wake-up time.

Light therapy can be used to treat patients with ASPS. In contrast to DSPS, however, the treatment for ASPS is administered in the evening to delay sleep onset. It is important to rule out depression, which is another cause of early morning awakening.

Shift work sleep disorder

If you work the night shift and typically go to sleep at 7 A.M. and wake up at 3 P.M., your body won't reset its clock when you have a weekend off to spend with people who work between 9 A.M. and 5 P.M. Drastic switches in bedtimes and wake times take a toll on the body and the brain, and people who suffer from shift work sleep disorder often feel in disarray.

Light exposure can help reset circadian clocks. It often is used in occupational settings to promote wakefulness outside of normal business hours. Similarly, keeping the bedroom dim at bedtime will promote sleep when the worker needs it. Workers should establish an environment free of distraction so they can sleep during the day.

Recently, Provigil received FDA approval for treating daytime sleepiness in shift workers. Shift workers with daytime sleepiness, insomnia, or impaired performance should consult their physician to rule out sleep disorders such as sleep apnea and periodic limb movements, which may be adding insult to injury.

Jet lag disorder

Jet lag occurs when insomnia or daytime sleepiness develops as a result of transmeridian jet travel across at least two time zones. Eastward travel that requires advancing sleep onset is more difficult to adjust to than westward travel, when sleep onset is delayed. Impaired functioning and physical symptoms like gastrointestinal upset are often present when someone is suffering from jet lag. Melatonin is often used to promote sleep so individuals with jet lag can reset their circadian clocks.

For best results and to reduce the chance of developing just lag, travelers should conform to the time zone of their destination and to avoid sleeping before it is dark. This is the best way to reestablish sleeping patterns and avoid severe daytime sleepiness.

Chapter 12

Sleep in Special Populations

People who say they sleep like a baby usually don't have one.

—Leo J. Burke

Sleeping habits start in the crib and change as we age. Parents usually establish the foundation for healthy habits that promote sleep. They introduce us to bedtime rituals, which might include a favorite storybook, a glass of warm milk, a nightlight, and the assurance that mom and dad are not far away.

As we grow older, our lifestyles evolve into a complicated web of school, friends, hobbies, relationships, careers, and emotional trials that inevitably interfere with our sleeping patterns. Illness, medications, and psychiatric problems can cloud our dreams and turn a good night into a nightmare. At every stage of life, there are obstacles to our pursuit of sound sleep.

How can we establish and maintain habits that will prepare us to obtain quality sleep throughout life? And in populations most vulnerable to change—particularly children and older adults—what are some signs of potential sleep disorders?

We know that sleep is critical to health at every age. We also know that children and older adults are more prone to certain sleep disorders, and these populations also experience sleep patterns that can be confused with disorders. In this chapter, we will identify:

- Ways to understand why sleep is so important for children and seniors
- What symptoms are normal signs of aging
- Symptoms that could indicate a sleep disorder

Children and Sleep

Sleep patterns change dramatically between birth and adolescence.

In the first few months of life, babies sleep between 12 and 18 hours over the course of a 24-hour day. Sleep periods last from minutes to hours and are interrupted by feedings and diaper changes.

During a child's first year, sleep becomes more consolidated at night and the number of naps during the day gradually decreases. Nighttime feedings fade away. By nine months of age, most babies sleep through the night. Infants typically sleep between 9 and 12 hours during the night and take naps that are between 30 minutes and 2 hours in duration, one to four times a day.

Children between 1 and 3 years of age require about 12 to 14 hours of sleep each day. By about 18 months of age, naps decrease to once per day and generally last an hour or two.

Preschoolers (age 3 to 5 years) typically sleep between 11 and 13 hours each night. By the time they reach the age of 4 or 5, most children no longer nap.

Between the ages 5 and 12, children need 10 to 11 hours of sleep each night. During the primary school years, sleep may begin to be short-changed as children juggle demands from homework and social activities, television, computers, and caffeine.

Teenagers require between 8.5 and 9.5 hours of shut-eye. High schoolers are particularly vulnerable to sleep deprivation because their circadian clocks shift to a later sleep time, keeping them feeling awake later in the evening hours.

See appendices 4 and 5 for quick guides to sleep in children and teens.

When sleep suffers, children:

- Forget what they learn in school
- Are grumpy and ornery
- Have difficulty concentrating during games or sports
- Show less patience with their siblings and friends
- Will "turn off" requests from teachers and parents, or have a tough time listening in general

By contrast, children who sleep well at night, and whose parents establish and enforce bedtime rituals, are more attentive, creative, and healthy. Ideally, sound sleep patterns start well before a child can communicate feelings of fatigue, hunger, or fear. If your child has sleep difficulties, remember that good sleeping habits or changes toward better sleeping habits take time. Your child will benefit from the structure you provide.

Check out Sleep for Kids, starring P.J. Bear, a service from the National Sleep Foundation, at *www.sleepforkids.org*. This interactive website teaches kids about what happens while we sleep through games and other activities. There's also a section for parents and teachers.

Don't all parents with children suffer from sleepless nights?

Parents are especially sensitive to the sounds of their upset children. When an infant fusses, a parent's natural reaction is to run to the crib to comfort the little one. But when this habit occurs every hour, every night, parents must take measures to improve sleep quality for the entire family.

Certain medical conditions, such as colic, might explain why an infant is agitated at night. Describe your child's sleep patterns to your pediatrician, who can provide advice on how many hours your baby should sleep each night and offer guidance to help your child establish nighttime sleep habits. Problems are often learned behavior and can be cleared up with a little advice from your doctor or other parents.

Remember, parents play the primary role in promoting sound sleep for their children. Just as we learn how to tie our shoes and ride a bike, we must learn how to sleep through the night. This is possible only when parents set boundaries.

How do I train my child to react to a healthy bedtime?

It is a scenario that is familiar to so many parents:

> *I can hear the rustling in the crib and the first hiccups of a night tantrum through the baby monitor before Emma starts a fit. I know I shouldn't go to her every time she cries, but I can't stand to hear her so unhappy. If I hold her and pace the nursery, she is usually asleep on my shoulder in ten minutes. The only problem is that this has become a routine and it happens every two hours all night long.*

Every person awakens for short periods of time during the night; we usually do not remember these awakenings because they are so brief. But infants and children can respond differently to nighttime arousals. They may feel insecure or frightened, and they express these emotions by crying.

Parents naturally want to comfort their baby. This becomes a problem when the child associates falling asleep with being held, walked around the room, rocked, or driven around the block. Rather than learning to fall asleep alone, the baby requires a parent's touch. Without this contact, the child experiences great difficulty falling back asleep.

To correct the problem, you must teach the baby to fall asleep without your help. If you typically "rescue" your child several times each night, a gradual approach is best. First, make sure there is something in the room to comfort your baby when you are not there. A CD player attached to the crib to play lullabies or a white-noise machine often does the trick. The point is to help your child associate sleep onset with something other than you.

When your baby cries at night, avoid immediate response. This can be more difficult for the parent than for the child, but by returning to the child's room seconds after fussing begins, you will re-teach the association you are trying to break.

The following technique might assist you over a six-month period to teach your child to fall asleep without your presence. First, tuck your child in as normal and say goodnight. (Remember that infants should always be put to bed on their backs; tummy-sleeping is associated with Sudden Infant Death Syndrome, or SIDS.) Leave the room, and be sure to allow a little light to enter the nursery. If your child begins to cry and is still crying after a few minutes, return to the room and comfort her with words or touching her back to convey safety and comfort. If your child continues to cry, wait a little longer before returning to the room, still resisting the temptation to pick up or hold her. On subsequent nights, return after progressively increasing intervals. After a few nights, parents usually see improvement. For more on this strategy and sleep in children, check out *Solve Your Child's Sleep Problems*, by Richard Ferber.

Curbing nighttime appetites Excessive nighttime feeding can also cause parents and children to lose sleep. Overfeeding translates to several awakenings during the night for infants and even one nightly feeding for babies 6 to 11 months old. Ask your pediatrician for more specific guidelines, as each child has different needs. Similar to sleep onset association, if parents feed their child several times during the night, the child's body might actually learn to be hungry at that time of night.

Not sure if your baby craves the bottle too much during the night? Check his or her diaper. A soaked diaper in the middle of the night might be an indication that a child is eating too much. If this is the case, gradually reduce the number of nighttime feedings. You can start by decreasing the quantity in the bottle or by waiting two hours between feedings the first night and gradually increasing times between feedings.

Set limits Toddlers can invent many creative reasons why parents should extend bedtime by reading just one more book or refilling a juice glass. A child may stall bedtime with special requests for hugs, tissues, or an urgent need to ask a parent an important question. *Will you turn the lights on? I'm scared when the door is closed. Can I sleep with you tonight? But I'm not tired . . . .* My five-year-old daughter's newest diversion attempt starts with *"Excuse me, Mama, but may I ask you a question?"*

Many parents struggle to say no when their children push bedtime limits. Perhaps the mother stayed at work late and feels she hasn't spent enough quality time with her son before tucking him in. What's one more story or another glass of water? Or maybe the father has been out of town for a few nights and feels missed when his daughter asks if he will stay in the bedroom until she falls asleep. Both parents' intentions are loving and natural. But neither parent is setting boundaries for their children or teaching that bedtime means preparing for sleep.

Quality time before bed is an important part of a nighttime ritual. Establish a routine with your children so you can spend quality time together—with limits.

The good sleep hygiene that promote sound sleep in adults is just as important for children and perhaps more so, as they are learning how to fall asleep on their own.

Bedtime ritual

Set a bedtime. If children know that 8 P.M. is when they should be under the covers—no exceptions for babysitters or caregivers—they will not protest when a parent starts the bedtime process.

Brush teeth, get ready for bed. Establishing basic habits will help set a routine for children so they associate a sequence of events with sleep.

Read a story. Winding down the evening with a storybook is a good way for parents to spend quality time with their children before bed. This routine also signals to children that it is quiet time. Just don't let one story turn into a book series. If children know that mom reads one book, or each parent reads one story, they will not bargain for a later bedtime.

Say goodnight. These words are a conclusion to the day—activities are over, time for bed. This verbal trigger lets children know that they must close their eyes and go to sleep.

Leave the room. Turn on a nightlight or keep a door cracked open if these conditions make your child feel more secure.

Do not:

- Substitute a television program for personal interaction
- Allow your child to fall asleep with a bottle or while being rocked or held
- Give your child drinks or food that contain caffeine or sugar before bed
- Participate in playful activity before bedtime

A word about teenagers Like younger children, teens are also prone to sleep problems, as highlighted by the 2006 National Sleep Foundation Poll. The survey found that, on average, adolescents get about seven and a half hours of sleep on school nights; the amount varies by grade, with teens tending to sleep less as they get older. An estimated 45 percent of adolescents are getting an insufficient amount of sleep on school nights and 31 percent get a borderline amount of sleep (eight to less than nine hours). This means that only 20 percent of adolescents are getting an adequate amount of sleep. Teens sleeping less on school nights are much more likely to feel sleepy, irritable, and depressed. They are also more apt to fall asleep in class and drink caffeinated beverages the next day. In addition, adolescents who get insufficient sleep are more likely than their peers to get lower grades. In contrast, the poll found that 71 percent of parents believe their teen gets enough sleep every night or almost every night. (See appendix 5, A Quick Guide to Teens and Sleep.)

Sleeping as We Age

A number of myths surround sleep and aging:

- *The more birthdays we celebrate, the more sleep we need.*
- *As we get older, sleep quality goes downhill.*
- *Activity is for kids; naps are for grandparents.*

The truth is that not one of these assumptions is true. Many seniors sleep about the same amount at age 65 as they did when they were younger—they just might not sleep those seven to nine hours during the same stretch of time. Some senior citizens find that the amount of sleep they need to feel refreshed is less than the amount they required in the past. Still others are dissatisfied with the changes that have occurred in their sleep patterns as they have aged and are looking for explanations.

It is perfectly normal for adults of any age to want to nap during the day; our bodies are wired based on circadian rhythms that tend to slow us down in late afternoon. Similarly, there is also no truth to the myth that activity is just for the kids. Active older adults who are engaged socially with family and friends, who are in high spirits, who exercise, and who maintain a positive outlook on life will experience less trouble falling asleep at night and fewer nighttime awakenings.

The myth that sleep quality deteriorates with age was debunked by the 2003 National Sleep Foundation poll, which reported that many older Americans actually sleep better than adults between the ages of 18 and 54. The study showed that 56 percent of older adults (ages 55 to 84) sleep an average of seven to nine hours, compared to 51 percent of younger adults who log that many hours.

Our sleep quality and quantity do change as we age, and it is important to distinguish between what is normal and what symptoms are signs of a sleep disorder.

What is normal sleep for mature adults? Just as each of us ages differently, our sleep patterns evolve as we age. Some people go gray sooner or retire into a more sedentary lifestyle, while others remain engaged and are just as active as their adult children. Some sleep often during the day and report restless nights. Others sleep fitfully, wake up energized, and notice that they need less sleep than they did when they were younger.

Certain changes are normal during the aging process, and being mindful of those changes allows sleep professionals to distinguish between maturation and the onset of a sleep disorder. A number of facts about sleep and aging are clearly established:

- Older people sleep about the same amount as they did when they were younger but are less likely to sleep during one stretch of time.

- Mature adults spend the same amount of time in REM sleep but spend less time in deeper stages of NREM sleep.

- Most people over the age of 65 awaken more often during the night.

- As we age, our internal sleep clocks, or circadian rhythms, take longer to adjust to changes. This can trigger sleep problems in people who travel frequently or who work irregular hours.

- Because older adults spend less time in deep sleep stages, they tend to be more sensitive to environmental disturbances, such as changes in temperature, light, and outside noise.

- Older adults might have a quiet, restricted lifestyle or sleep often during the day. Less active individuals tend to experience more difficulty sleeping at night simply because they are not as tired.

What changes in sleep are common as we age?

Because sleep quantity and quality changes as we age, older adults often complain of insomnia-related symptoms, such as waking frequently during the night or listening to the clock tick for hours before falling asleep.

Sometimes, age-related changes can disguise sleep disorders. About two-thirds of older adults surveyed in 2003 by the National Sleep Foundation say they experience one or more of the following symptoms at least a few nights each week:

- Difficulty falling asleep
- Waking often during the night
- Waking early and not being able to go back to sleep
- Feeling unrefreshed in the morning
- Snoring
- Pauses in breathing
- Unpleasant feelings in legs

Interestingly, only a fraction of survey respondents with these complaints said they had been diagnosed with a sleep disorder. One thing these older adults did have in common was their health. Eighty-five percent of those who rated their health as fair or poor reported sleep problems.

Does advanced age always bring about sleep problems?

A number of factors affect how we sleep as we age; some of them are medical, others are emotional. Less activity and general aches and pains keep some mature adults awake at night. Life changes, such as loss of a loved one, can also be responsible for disrupting sleep. A wife who has slept next to her husband for 40 years, and must retire to bed at night alone after his death, is likely to find that this difficult life transition inevitably inhibits her sleep.

Poor sleep also is associated with medical and psychiatric problems that may develop as we age. Illnesses can promote sleep disorders. Depression is known to disrupt sleep (and often parlays into insomnia). Chronic obstructive pulmonary disease, heart disease, and arthritis are often cited as the causes of sleep problems. Similarly, medications can prevent patients from falling or staying asleep, and even alterations in dosage or timing can affect sleep quality.

In addition to causing sleep problems, medical conditions can also disguise primary sleep disorders. In such cases, the frequent awakenings or daytime sleepiness that are hallmarks of many sleep disorders can be misinterpreted as a side effect of a medical condition. A patient afflicted with a medical condition and an undiagnosed sleep disorder might not respond to treatment for the medical problem, continuing to feel tired, irritable, or restless at night. Rather than considering that these symptoms indicate a primary sleep disorder, the patient simply assumes that he or she is sick and needs more medication or treatment.

Following are a handful of sleep disorders that present later in life. These conditions are not limited to mature adults, but are more likely to occur in older individuals than other sleep disorders.

Sleep apnea Sleep apnea disrupts breathing to varying degrees in one of four people over the age of 60. Primary symptoms are daytime sleepiness and snoring.

Wandering Confusion and wandering during the night is common among senior adults who live in long-term care facilities. This situation presents a catch-22 for caregivers who work in hospitals or nursing homes. To solve the problem, health workers may dispense sedative drugs to wanderers so they do not injure themselves or disturb other residents in the facility during the night. But some of these drugs promote confusion and increase the chance of falling. Seniors treated with them are at an increased risk of hip fractures sustained during nighttime strolls.

Drugs in the benzodiazepine class can produce disorientation outside the nursing home setting, too. For example, one doctor boarded a plane to South America, where he was slated to speak at an international medical convention. To offset jet lag, he took a benzodiazepine. Rather than arriving at his destination refreshed and ready for the conference, however, he accidentally deplaned during a connection when he was supposed to remain on the aircraft. He wandered the airport, completely confused. He was in the wrong country, which he didn't realize until he finally broke down and asked an attendant for help. He made it to the conference, but he arrived jet-lagged and too shaken from the experience to chance taking another benzodiazepine to counteract his jet lag.

Advanced sleep phase syndrome A pattern of "early to bed, early to rise" can develop as we age. In this case, *early* might mean well before 9 P.M., in which case rising occurs during hours when most adults are still asleep. People with advanced sleep-phase syndrome might awaken at 4 A.M. after sleeping for seven hours. This sleep schedule can inhibit a person from enjoying a fulfilling social life.

Patients with ASPS should try to stay awake later to postpone early morning awakenings. Exposure to daylight during the late afternoon can "trick" the body's internal clock into staying up later.

Periodic limb movement disorder About one-third of people over age 60 experience leg movement like twitching or muscle jerks during the night. These movements may cause arousal, which can affect the quality of sleep.

REM behavior disorder Most common in men over the age of 50, this disorder's primary symptom is that paralysis does not occur during REM sleep. As a result, an affected person can act out dreams, sometimes resulting in violent physical behavior that harms the patient or his bed partner. (Read more about this in chapter 10.)

How can I get a good night's sleep if I am an adult over age 50?

Sleep hygiene is just as important for mature adults as it is for younger people and children who are just learning healthy bedtime behavior. Because older individuals are sensitive to light, sound, and temperature during sleep, establishing an environment that promotes sleep is especially important. Among the steps recommended to maintain good sleep hygiene are to:

- Maintain regular wake times
- Go to sleep only when you are drowsy
- Use your bedroom only for sleep and intimate relations
- Avoid excessive daytime naps; if you nap, do so for no longer than one hour and not so late in the day that it interferes with your ability to fall asleep at night
- Stay active during the day
- Avoid large meals before bed
- Avoid nicotine and caffeine within six hours of bedtime
- Limit alcohol consumption
- Develop a bedtime ritual

Active days for restful nights Slowing down when you get older is natural, but stopping activity completely compounds sleep and other medical problems. Of course, *active* is a relative term. For some individuals, a quick walk around the block once a day is enough to tire their body and promote sleep at night. For others, activity is gardening, visiting with a friend or family member, or going to the store. Activity also includes mental pursuits: reading, writing a letter, knitting, or completing a crossword puzzle. For less mobile people, active may translate to simply staying awake rather than sleeping through one television program after the next.

Depending on how lively your mental and physical condition allows you to be, some level of activity is essential for maintaining overall health—and for sleeping soundly at night.

Chapter 13

Sleep Medicine Today

Sleep is the golden chain that ties health and our bodies together.

—Thomas Dekker

According to the 2005 Sleep in America poll conducted by the National Sleep Foundation (NSF), half of us sleep soundly and the other half, well, we're probably watching more late-night infomercials and counting far too many sheep to get those coveted hours of sleep we need. But the same poll uncovered some worrisome statistics: Troubled sleepers get into 60 percent more automobile accidents and are more likely to be diagnosed with high blood pressure, arthritis, heartburn, and diabetes than the well-rested bunch. What's more, 64 percent of nonsleepers are overweight. And many nonsleepers are too exhausted and frustrated to perform well at work or to function properly at home.

Sleep is not something to take for granted or to dismiss lightly. Rather, sleep is as important to the mind and body as drinking fluids to quench thirst and eating healthy food to alleviate hunger pangs. Sleep is a critical stop on the road to a healthy, happy life.

Today, more patients and physicians are recognizing the role sleep medicine plays in promoting overall wellness.

The Emergence of Modern Sleep Medicine

Sleep medicine is gaining more attention. Advances in research are sparking interest in the field, and its relevance to other specialties, from pediatrics to cardiology to bariatric surgery, is becoming increasingly clear. Sleep medicine is not an isolated island in the medical world—it is linked to every discipline because sleep affects our whole health. A record of disturbed sleep, daytime sleepiness, and problematic sleeping behavior such as snoring worsen preexisting medical problems and can interfere with treatment of those conditions.

Sleep medicine has begun to play a critical role in how doctors treat patients for other medical problems. In fact, a laundry list of diseases is linked to primary sleep disorders:

- Cardiologists are increasingly recognizing that nearly 50 percent of their patients might suffer from sleep apnea.

- Difficulty falling asleep, staying asleep, or awakening early in the morning are some of the most common presenting symptoms of mood disorders, such as depression or anxiety.

- Strong connections exist between REM behavior disorder and degenerative disorders affecting the nervous system, including Parkinson's disease.

- Restless legs syndrome is common among patients with anemia or low levels of iron, and also in patients with kidney failure.

- Children with attention deficit disorder are more likely to be diagnosed with obstructive sleep apnea.

- Partial sleep deprivation was recently shown to increase one's risk of developing Type 2 diabetes.

Now more than ever before, sleep specialists are identifying symptoms that emerge during sleep studies and interviews and might indicate the presence of other health problems.

Social issues are also linked to disrupted sleep. The list of normal day-to-day functions that are affected by a lack of sleep is sobering: an increase in occupational and motor vehicle accidents; a decline in academic achievement; an inability to carry on healthy relationships; and a diminished workplace performance.

Why are sleep studies on the rise?

Once a luxury test with a long waiting list, overnight sleep studies are becoming both more popular and a norm at medical institutions, which are building sleep labs and funding sleep medicine departments as patient demand continues to soar. Cleveland Clinic sleep experts test more than 150 patients each week in one on-site and seven off-site lab locations. The current statistics represent a tremendous jump from just over four years ago, when the one lab housed in the main medical facility tested 45 patients per week and the waiting list for an overnight study was six months long.

Why the demand? Why all the attention on sleep? And why are patients and insurance providers willing to pay for these tests?

Doctors attribute the surge in popularity to a media blitz prompted in part by society's wellness craze, but also by advances in sleep research, the results of which are reported in consumer magazines and other publications. Headlines about sleep have prompted us to think more seriously about the way sleep affects every part of our lives—not just our energy level during the day, but our risk of crashing our cars, our potential for gaining weight, and our ability to establish and maintain lasting relationships.

Doctors are conducting more overnight sleep studies in conjunction with assessments they perform for an array of health problems, but patients are asking for polysomnograms, too. The general public understands that not sleeping is a problem—one that we can solve if we turn to our doctors for help. The media tell us it's worth our time to catch some z's, and national health associations are confirming that fact with reports about how sleep affects our overall health.

Finding an accredited sleep lab You might think a sleep study is like a chest X ray—same test, different lab, no big deal. But this is not the case. If your doctor recommends a sleep center for your overnight study, you should double-check that the facility is accredited by the American Academy of Sleep Medicine. Some insurance companies decline coverage for studies that take place in unaccredited labs. Moreover, some labs specialize in studies of sleep apnea, while others offer a full menu of sleep services and may be more experienced handling other problems, such as narcolepsy, circadian

Insurance and Your Sleep Study

As a rule, insurance reimbursement for overnight sleep studies is not a problem for patients with sleep apnea or narcolepsy because both disorders are widely recognized as having adverse affects on health and performance. They are treatable and can be readily diagnosed with sleep laboratory testing.

A benefits request for an overnight sleep study to diagnose insomnia, the most common sleep complaint on the other hand, will prompt an insurance provider to take a second look at the claim. Most people with insomnia require a detailed sleep and medical history, but not necessarily an overnight sleep study. Only in severe cases in which sleep assessments and clinical testing have failed will sleep specialists order an overnight test for insomnia patients. The majority of insomnia cases can be treated with medications and behavioral therapy.

Beyond overnight sleep studies, insurance companies typically cover treatments such as continuous positive airway pressure therapy (when a patient is diagnosed with sleep apnea by a sleep study); certain medications; dental devices (though this depends on the provider and the diagnosis); and specific approved surgeries. Coverage always varies with provider and region.

rhythm disorders, and nocturnal seizures. Many labs have limited experience evaluating children and patients with special needs.

Many sleep centers, both affiliated with medical centers and independent, have websites that describe the services they offer. If you're not sure where to start, try

SleepCenters.org *www.sleepcenters.org*. This one lists sleep labs accredited by the American Academy of Sleep Medicine by zip code so you can search for the one closest to home.

Here are some other useful sites:

American Academy of Sleep Medicine *www.aasmnet.org*

SleepEducation.com *www.sleepeducation.com*

American Insomnia Association *www. americaninsomniaassociation.org*

American Sleep Apnea Association *www.sleepapnea.org*

Cleveland Clinic Sleep Disorders Center *www. clevelandclinic.org/neuroscience/treat/sleep*

Narcolepsy Network *www.websciences.org/narnet*

National Institutes of Health *www.nih.gov*

National Sleep Foundation *www.sleepfoundation.org*

Restless Legs Syndrome Foundation *www.rls.org*

Sleep Research Society *www.sleepresearchsociety.org*

Once you've found a sleep specialist and an accredited lab, chances are you're well on the way to a restful night's sleep.

Conclusion

No Substitute for Sleep

S o now you've joined the ranks of millions of Americans who are waking up to the dangers of sleep disorders. You've seen that what constitutes a good night's sleep varies from person to person. Seven hours of sleep may be a luxury to one person, and nine hours may be more suitable for you. With sleep, there simply is no standard. Sleep requirements change as you age, as your body progresses through various stages of life, and as you experience emotions that inevitably take their toll. The key to understanding your body's requirement for sleep is to recognize the signals your body sends when you've shortchanged yourself of this precious commodity.

There is a difference between periods of troubled sleep and symptoms of a serious sleep disorder. If daytime sleepiness, forgetfulness, irritability, or restless nights concern you or a loved one, I urge you to talk to your doctor. He or she may refer you to a specialist or to a sleep laboratory for testing. But if your doctor doesn't have the time to talk sleep, don't stop there. Many health care providers have not yet awakened to the benefits of prescribing sleep medicine in the correct circumstances. If yours is among them, it may be time for a change. Do not wait, as many do, until your problem lands you in the spare bedroom, out of school or work, or worse yet, without a driver's license. The time to act is now.

Our bodies are wired differently and our chemistry is unique and complex. As such, there is no single formula for sound sleep. Perhaps this is why we marvel over sleep—no matter how much we know, quite a bit remains a mystery. But the field of sleep medicine has come a long way. We now can identify normal sleep in a scientific sense, and we can recognize patterns in people who display abnormal sleep behavior. Doctors across the country are diagnosing and treating sleep disorders, and improving our overall health as a result. Sleep isn't a waste of time; your health today and tomorrow vitally depends upon getting enough of it. Your awareness of sleep's role in your path to wellness is the first step toward a lifetime of truly good nights.

So, here's to a good night's sleep.

Acknowledgments

For nearly 15 years, I have had the privilege of working with hundreds of physicians, nurses, technicians, administrative professionals, and other staff in the Cleveland Clinic Sleep Disorders Center and worldwide. Each and every one these professionals has been dedicated to solving sleep's secrets and improving the lives of people with sleep disorders. In addition to thanking them, I would like to thank the thousands of patients I've treated over the years who have taught me so much about sleep medicine and even more about what it means to be a good doctor.

I would like to thank Kristen Hampshire, a fabulous freelance writer in Cleveland whose funny and clever style helped frame the first *Cleveland Clinic sleep guide—Getting a Good Night's Sleep*

Finally, I wish to express my deepest thanks to my husband, Errol Schaefer; our daughter, Isabela; my father, Eugene Foldvary; and the rest of my family, whose love and support have been a constant in my life.

Appendix 1

A Quick Guide to Getting a Good Night's Sleep

Use your bedroom only for sleep and intimate relations. This means:

- Not watching television or even reading in bed
- Not eating in bed
- Definitely not working in bed

Essentially, your bedroom should be a calming oasis. Even an alarm clock can be a distraction. Try turning the clock so it faces away from you so you don't obsess about time while you're trying to fall asleep.

Avoid caffeine within four to six hours of bedtime. This includes:

- Coffee, tea, and soda
- Chocolate
- Over-the-counter wakefulness-promoting agents and some prescription drugs

If you suffer from insomnia, limit your intake of caffeinated beverages and avoid drinking caffeine after noon. Excessive caffeine use can lead to withdrawal symptoms, which can affect one's ability to sleep.

Avoid nicotine close to bedtime

Like caffeine, nicotine is a sleep-inhibiting stimulant. People who stop smoking might experience withdrawal symptoms at first, including sleeplessness, but once their body adjusts, they will find that they wake up less often and sleep more soundly at night. If you can't stop smoking entirely, avoid smoking in the evening and absolutely do not smoke during the night.

Do not drink alcoholic beverages within four to six hours of bedtime

Despite the notion that a nightcap is just the thing to bring about a good night's sleep, alcoholic beverages actually interfere with the body's ability to maintain deep sleep, which refreshes the body. Alcohol might induce sleep at first, but people who consume alcohol on a regular basis are likely to wake up frequently and often report feeling drowsy and sleep-deprived in the morning.

Avoid large meals; settle for a small snack before bedtime.

Full meals before bedtime can trigger heartburn and stomachache—two reasons to eat heavy meals at least four hours before going to sleep. A light snack, on the other hand, can promote sleep. Milk or cheese and crackers are good bedtime snacks.

In addition:

- Sleep only when you are drowsy.
- If you cannot fall or stay asleep, leave your bedroom and read or engage in a relaxing activity in another room.
- Do not allow yourself to fall asleep outside the bedroom; return to your bed to rest.

- Maintain regular wake times.

- Avoid napping during the day. (If you're extremely exhausted, limit naps to less than one hour, no later than 3 P.M.)

- Avoid strenuous exercise within six hours of going to sleep.

- Minimize light, noise, and extreme temperatures in the bedroom.

Appendix 2

A Quick Guide to Caffeine

Product	Serving size (oz)	Caffeine content (mg)
Coca-Cola	8	23
Diet Coke	8	31
Diet Pepsi	8	24
Dr Pepper (regular and diet)	8	25
Mountain Dew (regular and diet)	8	37
Red Bull	10	80
Starbucks coffee, venti	16	550
Starbucks coffee, grande	12	375
Starbucks coffee, tall	8	250
Iced tea	08	25

Appendix 3

Sleep Aids Most Commonly Requested
from drugstore.com*

Active Ingredients	Brand names
Acetaminophen and diphenhydramine hydrochloride	Extra Strength Acetaminophen PM; Extra Strength PM; Legatrin PM
Acetaminophen and diphenhydramine citrate	Excedrin PM
Aspirin and diphenhydramine citrate	Alka-Seltzer PM; Bayer PM
Diphenhydramine hydrochloride	Nytol; Simply Sleep; Sominex; Unisom SleepGels
Diphenhydramine hydrochloride and magnesium salicylate tetrahydrate	Doan's PM
Doxylamine succinate	Unisom Nighttime Sleep-Aid

* *Adapted from "Recent Advances in the Treatment of Insomnia," by Kumar Budur, M.D., Carlos Rodriguez, M.D., and Nancy Foldvary-Schaefer, D.O.,* Cleveland Clinic Journal of Medicine, *2007;74:21–26.*

Hyoscyamus niger, nux Moschata, Passiflora incarnata, Robinia pseudoacacia, Stramonium	Boiron Quietude
Natrum muriaticum, Lycopodium, Ignatia, Valeriana, Chamomilla, etc.	Moon Drops Vanilla Lozenges
Passiflora incarnata, Avena sativa, Humulus lupulus	Hylands Calms Forte
Strychnos ignatia, sea salt, kava, etc.	NaturalCare Anxiety Relief

Appendix 4

A Quick Guide to Children's Sleep

Here are some tips to establish healthy sleep habits for kids.

- **Maintain a consistent sleep schedule.** Your child's bedtime and wake-up time should be about the same every day, weekends included. A consistent wake-up time allows your child to feel sleepy in the evening, allowing for quicker sleep onset.

- **Exercise daily.** Have your child make exercise part of the daily routine. Incorporating exercise at a young age will help establish it as a daily life-long healthy practice.

- **Don't go to bed hungry.** Make sure your child doesn't go to bed hungry. Provide a light, healthy snack, such as a glass of milk, a piece of fruit, or cereal and milk. Avoid a heavy meal within one to two hours of bedtime because it can interfere with sleep.

- **Avoid caffeinated products.** Your child should avoid products that contain caffeine, particularly in the late afternoon and evening. Remember that caffeine is found in teas, some clear sodas, energy drinks, and chocolate.

- **Plan some quiet time before bed.** Before bedtime, help your child set aside up to an hour for calm, enjoyable activities, such as listening to quiet music or reading a book. Television watching, demanding homework, and computer gaming are off limits. The last 10 to 15 minutes of your child's day should be spent in the room where your child sleeps. Children should be put to bed awake so they learn to fall asleep themselves.

- **Preparing the bedroom for sleep.** Your child's bedroom should be quiet, comfortable (at a temperature below 75 degrees Fahrenheit), and dark (a nightlight is acceptable to calm children who are afraid of the dark). Resist the urge to put a television in your child's bedroom. Incorporate security objects, such as a special blanket or stuffed animal, into the bedtime routine. Use the bedroom for quiet time and sleeping only; do not use the bedroom for time-outs or punishment. At the end of the day, say goodnight to your child, turn off the bedroom light, and leave the room.

- **Pay attention at naptime.** The amount of time your child spends napping depends upon your child's age: newborns nap on and off all day; 2-year-olds may nap for a total of one to three hours each day, with the time spread over one or two naps; and 4- to 6-year-olds may not require a nap at all. Too many naps or long naps during the day can interfere with a child's ability to sleep well at night.

Appendix 5

A Quick Guide to Teens and Sleep

The National Sleep Foundation's 2006 Sleep in America poll focused on the sleep habits of America's adolescents. The poll found that teens, from grades 6 to 12, are not getting the sleep they need, and this lack of sleep gets worse as they progress through their teenage years.

The following suggestions can help your teen get the sleep his or her changing body needs:

- **Get enough sleep.** Teenagers need about nine hours of sleep each night to be fully alert during the day. But many teens find that the demands of school, after-school sport and social activities, and even work make this nearly impossible. Many try to catch up on sleep on the weekend. A better strategy is to maintain regular bed- and wake-up times on weekdays and weekends, and not vary the schedule by more than an hour.

- **Take a snooze.** Naps are fine if your teen likes to take them. However, naps should be limited to no more than 20 to 30 minutes and taken no later than the early afternoon. Napping too long or too late in the day makes it difficult to fall asleep at bedtime.

- **Get regular exercise.** Daily exercise will lead to better fitness and better sleep. Encourage your teen to participate in some type of physical activity for 30 to 60 minutes several times a week. However, exercise within 2 to 3 hours of bed-time should be avoided because it can make it difficult for a teen to fall asleep.

- **Limit caffeine intake.** Caffeine can disrupt sleep, so con-sumption of caffeinated products should be avoided in the late afternoon and evening. Remember that caffeine is found in some teas, clear sodas, energy drinks, and chocolate.

- **Don't go to bed hungry.** Make sure your teen doesn't go to bed hungry. Provide a light, healthy snack, such as a glass of milk, a piece of fruit, or cereal and milk. Avoid heavy meals within one to two hours of bedtime because they can interfere with sleep.

- **Don't smoke and avoid alcohol.** Nicotine is a stimulant and can disturb sleep. Every effort should be made to avoid smoking entirely, but teens who do smoke should avoid this activity within an hour or so of bedtime and during the night. Use of alcohol, sleeping pills, and other over-the-counter sleep aids can disrupt sleep, cause residual daytime sleepiness, and interfere with driving.

- **Set time aside to wind down before bed.** Have your teen set aside up to an hour of quiet time before bedtime every night. This time should be used for calm, enjoyable activ-ities, such as listening to quiet music or reading a book. Television watching, computer gaming, exercising, or demanding studying should be avoided right before bed-time. The last several minutes of quiet time may take place in the room where your teen sleeps, but the bed should be reserved for sleeping only.

- **Make the bedroom an inviting, relaxing environment.** Your teen's bedroom should be quiet, comfortable (at a temperature below 75 degrees Fahrenheit), dark, and free of distractions. Resist the urge to put a television or other electronics in your teen's bedroom.

- **Consult your teen's doctor.** Tell your teen's doctor if your teen has persistent difficulties falling or staying asleep, excessive daytime sleepiness, snoring, or unusual behaviors at night. These are signs of potentially serious sleep disorders that can affect your teen's mental and physical well-being, school performance, and ability to safely operate motor vehicles.

Index

About the Author

Nancy Foldvary-Schafer, DO, is director of the Sleep Disorders Center and Sleep Medicine Fellowship Program at the Cleveland Clinic. She is associate professor of medicine (neurology) at the Cleveland Clinic Lerner College of Medicine of Case Western Reserve University with joint appointments in the Cleveland Clinic Epilepsy Center and Women's Health Center. Certified by the American Board of Neurology and Psychiatry in Neurology and Clinical Neurophysiology, the American Board of Clinical Neurophysiology and the American Board of Sleep Medicine, she has treated patients with sleep disorders and epilepsy at the Cleveland Clinic since 1995. She has served as a lead investigator on numerous clinical trials and has written extensively on sleep and epilepsy.